Central Nervous System Peptide Mechanisms in Stress and Depression

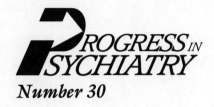

PROGRESS IN **PSYCHIATRY**
Number 30

David Spiegel, M.D.
Series Editor

Central Nervous System Peptide Mechanisms in Stress and Depression

Edited by
S. Craig Risch, M.D.

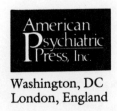

American Psychiatric Press, Inc.

Washington, DC
London, England

Note: The authors have worked to ensure that all information in this book concerning drug dosages, schedules, and routes of administration is accurate as of the time of publication and consistent with standards set by the U.S. Food and Drug Administration and the general medical community. As medical research and practice advance, however, therapeutic standards may change. For this reason and because human and mechanical errors sometimes occur, we recommend that readers follow the advice of a physician who is directly involved in their care or the care of a member of their family.

Books published by the American Psychiatric Press, Inc., represent the views and opinions of the individual authors and do not necessarily represent the policies and opinions of the Press or the American Psychiatric Association.

Copyright © 1991 American Psychiatric Press, Inc.
ALL RIGHTS RESERVED
Manufactured in the United States of America on acid-free paper.
First Edition
94 93 92 91 4 3 2 1

American Psychiatric Press, Inc.
1400 K Street, N.W., Washington, DC 20005

Library of Congress Cataloging-in-Publication Data

Central nervous system peptide mechanisms in stress and depression/edited by S. Craig Risch.—1st ed.
    p. cm.—(Progress in psychiatry; no. 30)
    Includes bibliographical references.
    ISBN 0-88048-249-4 (alk. paper)
    1. Affective disorders—Physiological aspects. 2. Stress (Physiology). 3. Corticotropin-releasing hormone.
4. Proopiomelanocortin. I. Risch, Samuel Craig. II. Series.
    [DNLM: 1. Corticotropin-Releasing Hormone—physiology. 2. Depressive Disorder—physiopathology. 3. Stress. Psychological—physiopathology. WM 171 C397]
RC537.C42 1991
616.85'2707—dc20
DNLM/DLC
for Library of Congress
                         90-14505
                            CIP

British Library Cataloguing in Publication Data

A CIP record is available from the British Library.

Contents

Contributors

Huda Akil, Ph.D.
Professor of Psychiatry, University of Michigan, Ann Arbor, Michigan

Jane M. Caudle, M.Ln.
Department of Psychiatry, Emory University School of Medicine, Atlanta, Georgia

Mary B. Eccard, R.N., M.S.
Clinical Nurse Specialist, Emory University School of Medicine, Atlanta, Georgia

James P. Herman, Ph.D.
Research Fellow, Department of Psychiatry, University of Michigan, Ann Arbor, Michigan

Michael Irwin, M.D.
Assistant Professor of Psychiatry, University of California at San Diego, San Diego, California

Rita D. Jewart, Ph.D.
Assistant Professor of Psychiatry, Coordinator, Clinical Research Program, Emory University School of Medicine, Atlanta, Georgia

Ned H. Kalin, M.D.
Professor of Psychiatry, University of Wisconsin Medical School, Madison, Wisconsin

Richard J. Lewine, Ph.D.
Associate Professor of Psychiatry, Emory University School of Medicine, Atlanta, Georgia

Juan F. López, M.D.
Research Fellow, Department of Psychiatry, University of Michigan, Ann Arbor, Michigan

Charles B. Nemeroff, M.D., Ph.D.
Professor of Psychiatry and Pharmacology, Duke University Medical Center, Durham, North Carolina

Michael J. Owens, Ph.D.
Fellow, Department of Psychiatry, Duke University Medical Center, Durham, North Carolina

William E. Pollard, Ph.D.
Assistant Professor of Psychiatry, Emory University School of Medicine, Atlanta, Georgia

Emile D. Risby, M.D.
Assistant Professor of Psychiatry, Emory University School of
Medicine, Atlanta, Georgia

S. Craig Risch, M.D.
Professor of Psychiatry, Director, Clinical Research Program, Emory
University School of Medicine, Atlanta, Georgia

Mark Stipetic, B.S.
Department of Psychiatry, Emory University School of Medicine,
Atlanta, Georgia

Lorey K. Takahashi, Ph.D.
Clinical Assistant Professor, University of Wisconsin Medical School,
Madison, Wisconsin

M. Adriana Vargas, M.D.
Research Analyst, Department of Psychiatry, Duke University
Medical Center, Durham, North Carolina

Stanley J. Watson, Ph.D., M.D.
Professor of Psychiatry, University of Michigan, Ann Arbor, Michigan

Elizabeth A. Young, M.D.
Assistant Professor of Psychiatry, University of Michigan, Ann Arbor,
Michigan

Introduction to the Progress in Psychiatry Series

The Progress in Psychiatry Series is designed to capture in print the excitement that comes from assembling a diverse group of experts from various locations to examine in detail the newest information about a developing aspect of psychiatry. This series emerged as a collaboration between the American Psychiatric Association's (APA) Scientific Program Committee and the American Psychiatric Press, Inc. Great interest is generated by a number of the symposia presented each year at the APA annual meeting, and we realized that much of the information presented there, carefully assembled by people who are deeply immersed in a given area, would unfortunately not appear together in print. The symposia sessions at the annual meetings provide an unusual opportunity for experts who otherwise might not meet on the same platform to share their diverse viewpoints for a period of 3 hours. Some new themes are repeatedly reinforced and gain credence, while in other instances disagreements emerge, enabling the audience and now the reader to reach informed decisions about new directions in the field. The Progress in Psychiatry Series allows us to publish and capture some of the best of the symposia and thus provide an in-depth treatment of specific areas that might not otherwise be presented in broader review formats.

Psychiatry is by nature an interface discipline, combining the study of mind and brain, of individual and social environments, of the humane and the scientific. Therefore, progress in the field is rarely linear—it often comes from unexpected sources. Further, new developments emerge from an array of viewpoints that do not necessarily provide immediate agreement but rather expert examination of the issues. We intend to present innovative ideas and data that will enable you, the reader, to participate in this process.

We believe the Progress in Psychiatry Series will provide you with an opportunity to review timely new information in specific fields of interest as they are developing. We hope you find that the excitement of the presentations is captured in the written word and that this book proves to be informative and enjoyable reading.

David Spiegel, M.D.
Series Editor
Progress in Psychiatry Series

Progress in Psychiatry Series Titles

The Borderline: Current Empirical Research (#1)
Edited by Thomas H. McGlashan, M.D.

Premenstrual Syndrome: Current Findings and Future Directions (#2)
Edited by Howard J. Osofsky, M.D., Ph.D., and Susan J. Blumenthal, M.D.

Treatment of Affective Disorders in the Elderly (#3)
Edited by Charles A. Shamoian, M.D.

Post-Traumatic Stress Disorder in Children (#4)
Edited by Spencer Eth, M.D., and Robert S. Pynoos, M.D., M.P.H.

The Psychiatric Implications of Menstruation (#5)
Edited by Judith H. Gold, M.D., F.R.C.P.(C)

Can Schizophrenia Be Localized in the Brain? (#6)
Edited by Nancy C. Andreasen, M.D., Ph.D.

Medical Mimics of Psychiatric Disorders (#7)
Edited by Irl Extein, M.D., and Mark S. Gold, M.D.

Biopsychosocial Aspects of Bereavement (#8)
Edited by Sidney Zisook, M.D.

Psychiatric Pharmacosciences of Children and Adolescents (#9)
Edited by Charles Popper, M.D.

Psychobiology of Bulimia (#10)
Edited by James I. Hudson, M.D., and Harrison G. Pope, Jr., M.D.

Cerebral Hemisphere Function in Depression (#11)
Edited by Marcel Kinsbourne, M.D.

Eating Behavior in Eating Disorders (#12)
Edited by B. Timothy Walsh, M.D.

Tardive Dyskinesia: Biological Mechanisms and Clinical Aspects (#13)
Edited by Marion E. Wolf, M.D., and Aron D. Mosnaim, Ph.D.

Current Approaches to the Prediction of Violence (#14)
Edited by David A. Brizer, M.D., and Martha L. Crowner, M.D.

Treatment of Tricyclic-Resistant Depression (#15)
Edited by Irl L. Extein, M.D.

Depressive Disorders and Immunity (#16)
Edited by Andrew H. Miller, M.D.

Depression and Families: Impact and Treatment (#17)
Edited by Gabor I. Keitner, M.D.

Depression in Schizophrenia (#18)
Edited by Lynn E. DeLisi, M.D.

Biological Assessment and Treatment of Posttraumatic Stress Disorder (#19)
Edited by Earl L. Giller, Jr., M.D., Ph.D.

Personality Disorders: New Perspectives on Diagnostic Validity (#20)
Edited by John M. Oldham, M.D.

Serotonin in Major Psychiatric Disorders (#21)
Edited by Emil F. Coccaro, M.D., and Dennis L. Murphy, M.D.

Amino Acids in Psychiatric Disease (#22)
Edited by Mary Ann Richardson, Ph.D.

Family Environment and Borderline Personality Disorder (#23)
Edited by Paul Skevington Links, M.D.

Biological Rhythms, Mood Disorders, Light Therapy, and the Pineal Gland (#24)
Edited by Mohammad Shafii, M.D., and Sharon Lee Shafii, R.N., B.S.N.

Treatment Strategies for Refractory Depression (#25)
Edited by Steven P. Roose, M.D., and Alexander H. Glassman, M.D.

Combined Pharmacotherapy and Psychotherapy for Depression (#26)
Edited by Donna Manning, M.D., and Allen J. Frances, M.D.

The Neuroleptic-Nonresponsive Patient: Characterization and Treatment (#27)
Edited by Burt Angrist, M.D., and S. Charles Schulz, M.D.

Negative Schizophrenic Symptoms: Pathophysiology and Clinical Implications (#28)
Edited by John F. Greden, M.D., and Rajiv Tandon, M.D.

Neuropeptides and Psychiatric Disorders (#29)
Edited by Charles B. Nemeroff, M.D., Ph. D.

Central Nervous System Peptide Mechanisms in Stress and Depression (#30)
Edited by S. Craig Risch, M.D.

Introduction

This volume summarizes new insights into the role of central peptidergic mechanisms (particularly corticotropin-releasing factor [CRF] and proopiomelanocortin [POMC]-derived peptides) in the pathophysiology of acute and chronic stress and in affective illness. During the past decade, there has been a virtual explosion of discoveries and integration of knowledge in this relatively new area of psychiatry. The contributors to this volume are leading neuroscientists whose past and ongoing major research efforts have been largely focused in this area. This volume describes research efforts spanning a continuum of technology from molecular biological/cellular to in vivo animal models and clinical studies in humans. The contributors attempt to delineate normal physiological and specific pathophysiological mechanisms in stress and depression. The authors address future directions of their own research efforts and the efforts of other investigators in the field. Thus, this volume not only summarizes current knowledge in the field, it also outlines the future directions of research efforts relevant to the field of psychiatry.

Drs. López, Young, Herman, Akil, and Watson eloquently and comprehensively summarize current knowledge about the normal physiology of the limbic hypothalamic-pituitary-adrenal (LHPA) axis. They also review studies delineating specific mechanisms in LHPA dysfunction in acute and chronic stress states and in affective illness. They emphasize the complexity of this system, indicating that multiple levels of both opposing and synergistic activities occur simultaneously both within single cells and neurons and at multiple anatomical levels of the organism. In particular, they describe fascinating studies suggesting that an individual responds to stress in the context of that individual's previous history of stress and his or her familiarity with the stressor. They describe molecular-biological techniques that have provided dramatic methodological advances to dissect and synthesize more adequately the complex interactions occurring simultaneously at many levels of this system.

Drs. Kalin and Takahashi describe a creative series of animal studies (in rats and rhesus monkeys) defining the role of CRF in adaptive and maladaptive responses to acute and chronic stress. They describe studies using CRF agonists and antagonists to produce "animal models" of depression and anxiety states that provide important linkage models to human illnesses. These animal models of human illness allow the investigation of specific mechanistic issues not currently possible in clinical studies in humans. Finally, they outline studies allowing insights into the normal and pathological "developmental" relationships between an organism's age (neonatal to adult), exposure, and response to acute and chronic stress.

Drs. Vargas, Owens, and Nemeroff synthesize their and others' studies of the role of central CRF mechanisms in the pathophysiology of depression. They summarize many studies that provide incontrovertible evidence for the mechanistic role of CRF in the pathophysiology of acute and chronic stress and depressive illness. Their studies have provided evidence for a direct mechanistic role of increased CRF neurotransmission in many of the pathological signs and symptoms associated with these disease states, including sleep and appetite disturbances, changes in autonomic and locomotor activity, and, more complexly, in memory and cognitive function. They also suggest evidence extending the mechanistic role of CRF into other human disease states including anorexia nervosa, Alzheimer's disease, and other neurodegenerative illnesses. They suggest the need for the development of novel pharmacological agents, including CRF agonists and antagonists, to treat or modulate these specific pathophysiological disturbances.

Our group summarizes our own studies, replicating the observations of Nemeroff and colleagues, of elevations in cerebrospinal fluid concentrations of CRF in severely depressed individuals. In ongoing efforts to further define the central nervous system (CNS) neurochemical mechanisms of central and peripheral alterations in LHPA-axis activity in depressed patients, we report the results of a research strategy using simultaneous assessments of CNS neurotransmitter activity and central and peripheral neuroendocrine activity. The results of our studies, to date, further emphasize the complexity of these systems and their interrelationships.

Dr. Irwin summarizes a rapidly expanding literature documenting immune disturbances associated with acute and chronic stress and with depressive illnesses. He describes his and others' studies of the role of 1) the hypothalamic-pituitary-adrenal axis, 2) central CRF mechanisms, and 3) endogenous opioid peptide mechanisms in the normal physiology of the immune system and in the pathophysiology of the immune system in specific disease states.

This volume summarizes exciting new insights into the role of CNS peptidergic systems (in particular the CRF-POMC system) in normal adaptive responses to stress and their potential dysfunction in maladaptive stress responses and in human disease states, particularly depression. More important, the contributors point toward the future directions of preclinical and clinical studies, which promise to result in novel and specific pharmacotherapies directed at modulating and/or correcting neuropeptide dysfunction in psychiatric illnesses.

Chapter 1

Regulatory Biology of the HPA Axis: An Integrative Approach

Juan F. López, M.D., Elizabeth A. Young, M.D.,
James P. Herman, Ph.D., Huda Akil, Ph.D.,
Stanley J. Watson, Ph.D., M.D.

The purpose of this chapter is to address the biochemistry and regulation of the hypothalamic-pituitary-adrenal (HPA) axis in depression in the context of brain-stress circuits. Basic animal research has provided new insights into how this neuroendocrine system is regulated at the cellular level and how the dynamics of the axis are reflected in peripheral and central changes during conditions of increased demand. Recent technical advances in the areas of neuroendocrinology and molecular biology have made it possible, for the first time, to begin to probe the circuits in the human brain that are responsible for endocrine control during stress. The HPA axis can be viewed as a hierarchical set of checks and balances with an ascending order of organization—from 1) specific gene products coding for hormones, transmitters, and receptors involved in the stress response, to 2) the individual cells, where the different molecules that participate in the stress response are synthesized, released, and regulated, to 3) neural circuits and endocrine components that integrate the complex sets of signals activated during stress—all of which operate across various time domains, in which the different components function and control the overall regulatory biology of the system. A knowledge of how this axis operates at the cellular, tissue, and system level is essential not only in interpreting the results of clinical psychoendocrinology studies, but also in designing new strategies to elucidate the role of specific central nervous system pathways in the neuroendocrine "alterations" found in depression. In this chapter, we focus on our current understanding of HPA regulation, derived from

This work was supported by NIMH grants MH-09632 (J.F.L.), MH-00427 (E.A.Y.), NS-08267 (J.P.H.), MH4-22251, and DA-02265 (H.A. and S.J.W.), by CRC grant 5M01-RR00042, and by a NARSAD grant (S.J.W.).

1

clinical and basic studies. We review the cell biology of peptide secretion and the neuroanatomical pathways that form the brain-stress circuit. We address the value of the chronic stress paradigm in interpreting results of clinical studies, including what circadian and feedback studies reveal about the level of regulation in the brain. Finally, we discuss how recent advances in neuroanatomy and molecular biology can help explore cellular regulation directly in brain and pituitary tissue, to understand the regulatory biology of the limbic system in stress and the relevance of these mechanisms to depression.

THE HPA AXIS AND DEPRESSION

The HPA axis is one of the central endocrine systems involved in the body's response to stress (Axelrod and Reisine 1984). Both physical and psychological stress trigger a neuroendocrine response that begins with several hypothalamic releasing factors, the most important of which are corticotropin-releasing hormone (CRH) and arginine vasopressin (AVP) (Antoni 1986; Jaeckle and López 1986). These hypothalamic factors trigger the release of the proopiomelanocortin (POMC)-derived peptides β-endorphin and ACTH from the anterior pituitary. In turn, ACTH stimulates the adrenal cortex to secrete glucocorticoids (cortisol in humans, corticosterone in rats). Circulating glucocorticoids interact with the hippocampus, hypothalamus, and pituitary by binding to glucocorticoid (type II) and mineralocorticoid (type I) receptors, to negatively regulate the axis by inhibiting subsequent release of ACTH (Keller-Wood and Dallman 1985; Sapolsky et al. 1986). In this manner, the axis forms a closed-loop feedback system that tightly regulates plasma glucocorticoid levels (Figure 1-1).

This regulation of glucocorticoid secretion during stress is critical for the survival of the organism. The absence of glucocorticoids leads to the inability of the organism to cope with stress and subsequent death (Bethune 1989). However, diseases of glucocorticoid excess, such as Cushing's and depression, make it clear that hypersecretion is also deleterious (Nelson 1989; Sapolsky et al. 1986). Therefore, the system is geared to maintain adequate glucocorticoid levels through an elaborate set of checks and balances.

There is a body of psychoendocrine research suggesting that the HPA axis is overstimulated in depressive illness (Kathol et al. 1989). The original studies of Sachar et al. (1973) showed that depressed patients demonstrated increased cortisol secretory activity as measured by plasma cortisol levels, the number of cortisol secretory episodes, and the number of minutes of active secretion. Later studies have continued to validate the hypercortisolemia of depression (Carroll et al. 1976a, 1976b; Halbreich et al. 1985; Linkowski et al. 1987; Pfohl et al. 1985a; Rubin et al. 1987). Studies by Carroll et al. (1976b, 1981) focused on the feedback elements of the HPA axis in depression using dexamethasone, a synthetic steroid that suppresses cortisol secretion for 24 hours in most normal controls. Following dexamethasone administration, some depressed patients who do not appear to be hypercortisolemic will show either a failure to suppress plasma cortisol or early escape from dexamethasone suppression. This failure to suppress cortisol with dexamethasone was interpreted as excessive central nervous system (CNS) drive to the pituitary from hypothalamic and limbic structures, particularly in the late afternoon and evening, a usually quiescent time for the HPA axis (Carroll et al. 1976a; Pfohl et al. 1985a). The "escape" from dexamethasone suppression was caused by a continued drive to the axis during the normal silent time of the circadian rhythm.

It was expected that the increased cortisol would be accompanied by an increased level of ACTH in plasma; however, this expectation has been difficult to validate because of apparent contradictory find-

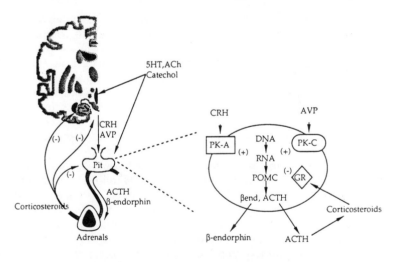

Figure 1-1. Primate hypothalamic pituitary adrenal axis (*left*) and pituitary corticotroph (*right*), showing regulatory events involved in ACTH synthesis and secretion. 5HT, serotonin; ACh, acetylcholine; Catechol, catecholamines; CRH, corticotropin-releasing hormone; AVP, arginine vasopressin; Pit, anterior pituitary; PK-A, protein kinase A; PK-C, protein kinase C; POMC, proopiomelanocortin; GR, glucocorticoid receptor; +, stimulation; −, inhibition.

ings in the studies that have addressed this issue. Several groups have demonstrated some differences in peptide responses (ACTH and/or β-endorphin) to dexamethasone (either between depressive and control subjects or within depressed patients) between dexamethasone cortisol suppressors and nonsuppressors (Berger et al. 1985; Holsboer et al. 1983; Kalin et al. 1982; Matthews et al. 1986; Nasr et al. 1983; Norman et al. 1987; Reus et al. 1982; Risch 1982; Winokur et al. 1985). Other studies, however, have found no peptide differences between depressives and controls or no correlation between steroid and ACTH responses (Beresford et al. 1985; Cohen et al. 1984; Fang et al. 1981; Rupprecht et al. 1988; Yerevanian and Woolf 1983). In a modification of the basic design, Yerevanian et al. (1983) showed that the postdexamethasone ACTH levels measured after recovery were higher in dexamethasone nonsuppressors than in suppressors. Risch (1982) explored the cholinergic link in the HPA hyperactivity and found β-endorphin hypersecretion in depression and schizoaffective disorder after physostigmine, compared to normal subjects and psychiatric control subjects, suggesting cholinergic hyperactivity in affective disease.

In general, these basal and postdexamethasone studies do not lead to a consistent picture. The results are difficult to compare, partly because of different study designs and variability of the radioimmunoassays but also probably because of the intrinsic variation of HPA function in the populations studied. If depressed patients can exhibit multiple patterns of response to dexamethasone as a function of their clinical or endocrine history, then comparing group means—for example, depressive subjects versus normal subjects—will not likely indicate a significant difference, unless the depressive group is extremely homogeneous or the number per group is quite large. Another explanation for the inconsistency could be found in the fact that some studies compared plasma ACTH following dexamethasone of cortisol suppressors with that of nonsuppressors, sometimes without normal controls (Rupprecht et al. 1988; Winokur et al. 1985; Yerevanian et al. 1983), or compared endogenous and nonendogenous depression (Rupprecht et al. 1988). Preselecting a comparison of pituitary peptides based on cortisol response to dexamethasone presupposes a consistency of the pituitary adrenal interface that may not always exist, because there are several tissue levels of regulation in the HPA axis. Hence, there is a need to devise criteria for normal or abnormal pituitary responses that can be applied at the level of the individual patient, as opposed to contrasting means (Matthews et al. 1986).

Some studies have investigated the circadian pattern of ACTH in depressed patients. Pfohl et al. (1985a, 1985b) were able to demonstrate small differences between normal control subjects and depressed subjects in their mean 24-hour plasma ACTH level. Linkowski et al. (1985, 1987) also found increased mean 24-hour ACTH as well as an earlier ACTH nadir in depressed patients: These changes were reversed after antidepressant treatment (Linkowski et al. 1987). This slight increase of plasma ACTH in depressed subjects is amplified to higher cortisol levels by the adrenal. Several studies have shown adrenal hypertrophy and enhanced response to ACTH in depressed subjects (Amsterdam et al. 1983; Dorovini-Zis and Zis 1987; Jaeckle et al. 1987).

It is not surprising that greatly elevated plasma ACTH levels have not been found in depressed patients. We know from animal studies that secretion is only the end point of several cellular and biochemical events, and peptide plasma levels do not necessarily reflect events occurring in the pituitary and brain (Akil et al. 1985; Shiomi et al. 1986). There are several regulatory events that occur within the cells at each tissue level (Figure 1-1). For example, in the pituitary corticotroph (the ACTH-producing cell), binding of a CRH molecule to its receptor produces a cascade of events that include production of new messenger RNA (mRNA) molecules (transcription), translation into protein (e.g., POMC, the precursor of ACTH and β-endorphin), processing of the precursor into the final products, accumulation of the peptides in secretory vesicles, and release of the peptides to the circulation. Studies in rodents have shown that CRH binding simultaneously leads to secretion and increases in transcription. On the other hand, glucocorticoids simultaneously control secretion of POMC and negatively control transcription (Lundblad and Roberts 1988). Therefore, when we look at plasma levels, we are looking at the net effect of two opposing stimuli in a closed-loop system, and studying the cellular components at each level of the system becomes necessary to understand regulation. Thus, a knowledge of the biochemistry of the cell and its elements is critical in understanding the biology of the system and the regulatory events that operate to produce or inhibit secretion during times of increased demand.

CELL BIOLOGY OF THE CORTICOTROPH

The cellular events that occur in the cortiotroph after the binding of a ligand to its receptor have been well studied both in pituitary tissue cultures and using tumor cell lines (Abou-Samra et al. 1987; Bilezikjian and Vale 1983; Lundblad and Roberts 1988; Miyazki et al. 1984; Perrin et al. 1986). Several molecules have been identified as capable of acting directly in the corticotroph to stimulate ACTH release, including epinephrine, norepinephrine, oxytocin, and angiotensin II; however, CRH and AVP seem to be the most important factors that stimulate secretion (Antoni 1986). CRH interacts with specific CRH receptors in the corticotroph cell membrane (Leroux and Pelletier 1984; Perrin et al. 1986). These receptors are coupled to adenylate cyclase through a guanine nucleotide binding protein, and binding of a CRH molecule stimulates secretion by increasing intracellular levels of cAMP and subsequent activation of protein kinase A (Aguilera et al. 1983; Perrin et al. 1986). CRH receptor binding in the pituitary has been reported to downregulate with in vivo maneuvers that increase endogenous CRH secretion, such as adrenalectomy and stress (De Souza et al. 1985; Hauger et al. 1988), although this does not necessarily mean that further stimulation of CRH will result in decreased releasability of POMC peptides (Young and Akil 1985).

AVP also acts through specific cytoplasmic membrane receptors, which respond predictably to in vivo maneuvers (Koch and Lutz-Bucher 1985). This vasopressin receptor, which is similar to the V_1-type receptor, is linked to the phosphatidyl inositol system and stimulates secretion through mobilization of intracellular calcium and activation of protein kinase C (Figure 1-1; Baertsch and Friedli 1985; Raymond et al. 1985). The fact that CRH and AVP act through different intracellular pathways may explain the synergistic effects on ACTH release that these two peptides have when administered concomitantly in vivo (Lamberts et al. 1984).

The specific cellular processes by which receptor activation results in activation of POMC gene expression are not well understood and probably involve *cis*-acting factors interacting with the 5' (promoter) region of the POMC gene, as has been shown for various other genes (McKnight and Kingsbury 1982; Scheidereit et al. 1986). Nevertheless, several in vitro experiments have shown that the cellular pathways involved in peptide secretion also stimulate transcription (Dave et al. 1987; Hollt et al. 1986; Loeffler et al. 1985; Reisine et al. 1985; Shiomi et al. 1986). The first product of the transcription of the POMC gene is a heteronuclear messenger RNA (hnRNA). This primary transcript contains two introns, which are rapidly spliced to form a mature POMC mRNA molecule (Affolter and Reisine 1985; Fremeau et al. 1986). The mature mRNA is then transported from the nucleus to the cytoplasm, where it will become part of the total mRNA pool, and can be translated in the ribosomal apparatus into several POMC polypeptide chains. Because the primary transcript is converted rapidly to mRNA, quantification of hnRNA is a good indication of transcriptional activity (i.e., de novo synthesis of mRNA).

Translation of the POMC mRNA produces a precursor molecule that, after maturation, gives rise to several biologically important products, including the stress hormone ACTH and the potent opioid β-endorphin (Figure 1-2). Although different cells in the body express the POMC precursor, the final products that are stored and secreted are quite different depending on the type of cell (Akil et al. 1981; Dores et al. 1986). This is due to tissue-specific processing. In the case of the anterior pituitary corticotroph, proteolytic cleavage at double basic residues gives rise to β-lipotropin, ACTH, and a 16-kilodalton N-terminal peptide. A percentage of the β-lipotropin and N-terminal peptide is further processed into β-endorphin and joining peptide, respectively. These different products are stored in secretory vesicles and later coreleased into the circulation. The relative amounts of peptide forms stored and released by endocrine cells and neurons can be significantly changed by various manipulations, apparently because of differential effects on the various enzymes involved in the pathway. Therefore, it is possible for a given cell to secrete a different mix of POMC products at different times, as a function of the demand for biosynthesis and release (Akil et al. 1985; Shiomi et al. 1986). This is a type of plasticity that has not been extensively explored and that represents an important aspect of the regulatory dynamics of the cell.

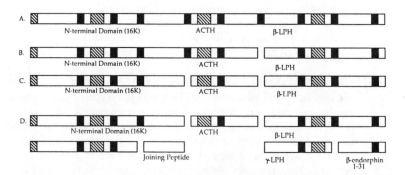

Figure 1-2. Proopiomelanocortin (POMC) structure and processing in anterior pituitary. *A*: Intact POMC molecule has molecular weight of 31 kilodalton. *B* and *C*: Proteolitic cleavage between two basic amino acids gives rise to β-lipotropin (β-LPH), ACTH, and a 16-kilodalton N-terminal fragment. These steps are common to all POMC-containing neuroendocrine tissues. *D*: Final products in anterior pituitary corticotroph are combination of partially and fully processed POMC peptides.

Another important aspect of corticotrophic cell regulation is the inhibitory action of glucocorticoids. In addition to controlling POMC gene expression through its effects at suprapituitary sites, in vitro studies have demonstrated that glucocorticoids also control POMC gene expression by acting directly at the corticotroph level (Eberwine et al. 1987; Nakamura et al. 1978; Roberts et al. 1979a, 1979b). This effect seems to be operative only in situations of prolonged corticotroph activation, because decreases of POMC mRNA levels are seen only after several hours of dexamethasone treatment (Nakamura et al. 1978; Roberts et al. 1979b). The precise molecular mechanism of this inhibition is not known, although it has been suggested that glucocorticoid receptors suppress transcription by interfering with the ability of an endogenous transcription factor to bind to a promoter DNA sequence of the POMC gene (Drouin et al. 1985).

Therefore, it is clear that at any one point, POMC synthesis and release lie at the nexus of the opposing influences of the feed-forward effects of secretagogues that activate biosynthesis and release and the feedback effects of steroids that inhibit these events. An additional level of complexity is given by the fact that cellular events that control biosynthesis and secretion are also occurring within each different tissue that is part of the HPA axis (Herman et al. 1989c). Thus, communication between the different components of the axis serves to transmit regulatory information so that it can be integrated into a coordinated physiological response. The brain circuits responsible for this integration form a complex network of checks and balances. Understanding the specific roles of these circuits has been one of the major tasks of regulatory neuroanatomy for the past decade.

NEURAL CIRCUITS REGULATING HPA FUNCTION

Most conceptual views of the HPA axis portray a system capable of executing rapid and efficient endocrine responses under conditions requiring adaptive behaviors on the part of the organism in question. Clearly, the execution of these responses is the province of the brain. In the wake of the discovery of CRH by Vale et al. (1981), it has become possible to definitively pinpoint parvocellular neurons of the hypothalamic paraventricular nuclei (PVN) as the prime movers of adrenocortical activation. Various immunohistochemical and lesion studies in rodents have revealed that PVN CRH neurons synthesize and supply CRH (as well as AVP) to the adenohypophysial circulation and are responsible for basal and stimulated release of ACTH (Antoni et al. 1983; Bruhn et al. 1984; Makara et al. 1981; Whitnall et al. 1987a). As such, these neurons constitute a final common pathway for ACTH release. However, the mechanism whereby the brain translates stimuli into the final integrated response at the PVN, and how this translation is muddled under chronic stimulation and pathological conditions, is presently ill-understood. Vital to this understanding is a knowledge of basic circuits contributing to HPA activation, inhibition, and negative feedback regulation by glucocorticoids and/or ACTH. In the following paragraphs, we briefly explore the status of what is known concerning HPA-relevant circuits, drawing heavily from recent studies performed in our laboratory.

The Hypothalamic PVN as Integrator of the HPA Response

Since the mid-1960s it has been known that the medial hypothalamus plays an important role in integration of the adrenocortical response. Numerous lesion studies have determined that damage to the medial basal hypothalamus causes marked deficits in adrenocortical responsiveness to various stressors. In the wake of the discovery of CRH, it has become clear that the primary locus of hypophysiotrophic activity in the brain is in the hypothalamic paraventricular nucleus. Using antibodies against CRH, numerous anatomical studies demonstrate a clear CRH-containing pathway projecting from the medial parvocellular subdivision of the PVN directly onto the vasculature of the external lamina of the median eminence (Antoni et al. 1983; Merchenthaler et al. 1983; Swanson and Sawchenko 1983). Subsequent physiological studies revealed an alarming specificity of hypophysiotrophic activity to this nucleus: Ablation or disconnection of this nucleus effectively blocks initiation of stress responses in vitro and in vivo (Bruhn et al. 1984; Makara et al. 1981). Further anatomical analysis of this well-defined region indicates that in addition to production of CRH, this nucleus also contains neurons synthesizing vasopressin, oxytocin, and angiotensin II (Kiss 1988), all of which show some ability to release ACTH from corticotrophs, either alone or in conjunction with CRH (Negro-Vilar et al. 1987; Plotsky 1987a, 1987b). These findings suggest that the PVN is in a position to influence ACTH release not only by secretion of CRH but also by secretion of other secretagogues.

One of the striking findings to emerge from anatomical studies of the PVN is coexpression of CRH with other ACTH secretagogues, most notably vasopressin, within the same neuron. Under normal conditions, CRH and AVP are segregated within the PVN, with AVP localized within magnocellular neurons of the posterior magnocellular PVN and CRH to parvocellular cells within the immediately adjacent, yet anatomically distinct, medial parvocellular region. In response to adrenalectomy, which removes circulating steroids and effectively opens up all glucocorticoid negative-feedback loops, the medial parvocellular PVN shows a marked increase in number and intensity of both CRH- and AVP-staining neurons (Kiss et al. 1984a; Sawchenko et al. 1984). The change in the number of detectable AVP neurons is quite striking, as few AVP-positive neurons can be seen in normal rats (Kiss et al. 1984a; Sawchenko et al. 1984; Whitnall 1988; Whitnall et al. 1987b). Colocalization studies further revealed that a substantial portion of CRH-positive neurons also stain for AVP, indicating synthesis of both secretagogues within the same neuron. Elegant work from Whitnall's laboratory has colocalized CRH and AVP to the same neurosecretory endings in the external lamina of the median eminence, furthering the notion of CRH and AVP cosecretion (Whitnall et al. 1987a). The percentage of terminals containing both CRH and AVP rises dramatically with physiological demand (adrenalectomy; Whitnall et al. 1987b), supporting the hypothesis of coordinate regulation of ACTH secretion by multiple secretagogues within the same neuron.

The advent of in situ hybridization technology has allowed characterization and quantitation of ACTH-secretagogue mRNA in the PVN under basal and stimulated conditions, allowing inferences to be drawn regarding biosynthesis of secretagogues under various conditions. Data from our laboratory and others have verified the presence of CRH mRNA at the level of the medial parvocellular PVN and have shown the expected up-regulation, ranging from twofold to threefold, of the CRH message in response to adrenalectomy (Harbuz and Lightman 1989; Schäfer et al. 1987; Young et al. 1986) or metyrapone treatment (S. Kwak, E. Young, P. Patel, 1988, unpublished observations). Examination of AVP mRNA in the medial parvocellular region indicated only background levels of AVP message in normal animals. Adrenalectomy, as expected, vastly increased AVP mRNA in this region some eightfold (Schäfer et al. 1987), verifying de novo synthesis of peptide in the face of steroid removal.

Analysis of the effects of stress on ACTH secretagogues revealed an interesting pattern of results. Our laboratory has demonstrated that chronic electroconvulsive shock treatment, which acts to up-regulate the HPA axis, results in a slight but significant up-regulation of CRH mRNA in the medial parvocellular PVN, without any change in AVP message. Interestingly, increased PVN CRH mRNA levels were accompanied by decreases in PVN CRH content, suggesting a more rapid turnover of CRH in response to the effective stimulus. These data demonstrate that chronic stress-induced HPA up-regulation may be mediated primarily by CRH, without a significant AVP component (Herman et al. 1989c). The efficacy of stress as an inducer of CRH mRNA is further indicated by studies using other chronic or acute stressors, including hypertonic saline (Harbuz and Lightman 1989; Lightman and Young 1987) and foot shock (Imaki et al. 1988). In all cases, one fact stands clear: CRH production is increased under conditions of chronic stress, even in the face of elevated corticosterone levels. These data suggest either resistance of the CRH neuron to results of glucocorticoid negative feedback or consistent drive of the HPA axis from some neuronal source.

In addition to affecting secretion of CRH and ancillary secretagogues in response to stress or physiological challenge, the PVN is also responsible for normal daily fluctuations in CRH activity. CRH mRNA levels in the PVN show significant circadian variation, being at their highest before initiation of the evening corticosterone rise in the rat (S. Kwak, E. Young, H. Akil, S. Watson, 1989, unpublished observations; Watts and Swanson 1989). Accordingly, ACTH-releasing activity of PVN extracts is highest during the corticosterone peak (Ixart et al. 1987; Szafarczyk et al. 1980b).

Anatomical Connectivity of the PVN

Knowledge of inputs to the PVN region can provide a good resource for examination of neuronal influences on the HPA axis. Given the importance of this region in HPA function as well as other endocrine and autonomic processes, much information has been gathered regarding connectivity of this nucleus. The general consensus of these data indicates that the medial parvocellular PVN receives direct afferents from a restricted set of brain nuclei, including the ventrolateral medulla, nucleus of the solitary tract, dorsal raphe nucleus, and nucleus raphe magnus in the brainstem; numerous hypothalamic nuclei, the most prominent of which are the suprachiasmatic nucleus, dorsomedial nucleus, arcuate nucleus, ventromedial nucleus, lateral hypothalamus, and median, medial, and lateral preoptic areas; the bed nucleus of the stria terminalis; the subfornical organ; and the medial and central amygdaloid nuclei (Gray et al. 1989; Sawchenko and Swanson 1983; Ter Horst and Luiten 1987). Among identified neurotransmitter/neuropeptide inputs from these regions are norepinephrine, epinephrine, and neuropeptide Y from medullary sites (Sawchenko et al. 1985); serotonin from the raphe nuclei (Sawchenko et al. 1983); ACTH from the arcuate hypothalamus (Kiss et al. 1984b; Piekut and Joseph 1985); and angiotensin II from the subfornical organ (Lind et al. 1985). Interestingly, Silverman et al. (1989) indicated the presence of CRH-positive nerve terminals in the medial parvocellular PVN, suggesting a CRH-containing input to the PVN and raising the intriguing possibility that CRH regulates its own release as a neurotransmitter. Several nuclei are candidates for this innervation, including the preoptic area, lateral hypothalamus, medial and central amygdala, and bed nucleus of the stria terminalis. Determination of the appropriate source awaits further analysis.

Although the connectivity of the PVN provides a basis for study of its physiological relationships with the rest of the brain, it does not totally predict spheres of influence on PVN neurons. Analysis of the physiological data clearly indicates that regions at least one synapse removed from the PVN are capable of influencing HPA function.

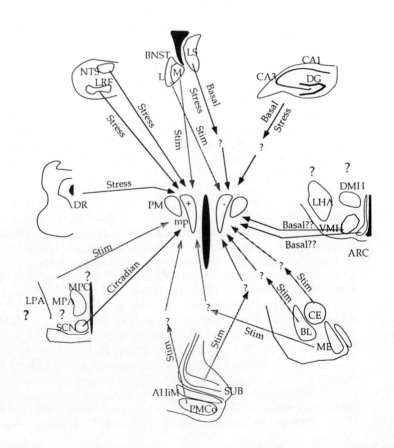

From this, it is clear that anatomical relationships of PVN need to be defined in multisynaptic terms as well as by projectional anatomy.

Pathways Involved in Activation of the HPA Axis

Studies from several laboratories indicate that release of CRH and ACTH can be affected via ascending inputs to the PVN (some of which are illustrated schematically in Figure 1-3). General disconnection of ascending afferents to the PVN regions by hypothalamic or midbrain knife cuts produces neuronal and endocrine sequelae in-

Figure 1-3. Some major brain regions influencing hypothalamic-pituitary-adrenal (HPA) function in the rat, with some attention paid to their anatomical relationship to the medial parvocellular paraventricular nucleus (PVN). The PVN occupies the center of the diagram. Inputs believed to be excitatory to corticotropin-releasing hormone (CRH) secretion and/or synthesis are designated by arrows projecting to left PVN; inputs believed to be inhibitory are designated by arrows projecting to right PVN. The word *basal* next to an arrow indicates that that projection influences basal function of the CRH neuron, *stress* indicates it is involved in stress regulation of the CRH neuron, and *circadian* indicates that the circuit is involved in circadian regulation of CRH neuron function. *Stim* indicates that stimulation of the indicated structure has effects on CRH neurons or HPA function; these arrows are shaded to distinguish electrical stimulation from physiological studies. Question marks between two arrows indicate that a synapse is likely to intervene between the originating structure and the PVN. Large question marks beside hypothalamic regions indicate that the regions' physiological relationship to PVN CRH neurons is largely unexplored. PM, posterior magnocellular PVN; mp, medial parvocellular PVN; NTS, nucleus of the solitary tract; LRF, lateral reticular formation; DR, dorsal raphe; LPA, lateral preoptic area; MPO, median preoptic nucleus; MPA, medial preoptic area; SCN, suprachiasmatic nucleus (hypothalamus); AHiM, amygdalohippocampal area, medial part; PMCo, posteromedial cortical amygdala; SUB, ventral subiculum; ME, medial amygdala; BL, basolateral amygdala; CE, central amygdala; ARC, arcuate nucleus of the hypothalamus; VMH, ventromedial nucleus of the hypothalamus; DMH, dorsomedial nucleus of the hypothalamus; LHA, lateral hypothalamic area; CA1, cornu ammonis 1 (pyramidal cell layer of the hippocampus); CA3, cornu ammonis 3 (pyramidal cell layer of the hippocampus); DG, dentate gyrus; LS, lateral septum; BNST, bed nucleus of the stria terminalis, medial (M) and lateral (L) divisions.

dicating impaired HPA activation, including dampening of corticosterone responses to sensory stimulation (Siegel et al. 1980), decreased corticosterone and ACTH responses to anesthesia and thoracotomy (Herman et al. 1990), and accumulation of CRH peptide in parvocellular PVN neurons (Sawchenko 1988). Attempts to localize excitatory inputs have succeeded in pointing out several brainstem loci involved in HPA activation. Noradrenergic and adrenergic neurons of the A1, A2, C1, and C2 regions of the caudal medulla, which send direct projections to the parvocellular PVN (Sawchenko et al. 1985), stand out as activators of the HPA axis. Numerous lesion studies (Alonso et al. 1986; Mezey et al. 1984; Szafarczyk et al. 1988) and pharmacological studies (Gibson et al. 1986; Plotsky 1987; Szafarczyk et al. 1987) clearly indicate a stimulatory action of these neuronal cell groups on CRH, ACTH, and corticosterone release, which appear to act via α-1 adrenoreceptors. The nucleus of the solitary tract, which encompasses but does not define the A2 (C2) region, is clearly involved in promoting release of ACTH in response to hypotension (Darlington et al. 1986). In addition, some evidence suggests that serotonin neurons of the pontine dorsal raphe nucleus and nucleus raphe magnus, which project to the parvocellular PVN (Sawchenko et al. 1983), are involved in HPA activation. Destruction of dorsal raphe 5-HT neurons diminishes the corticosterone response to neuronal stimulation (Feldman et al. 1987) and appears to dampen the circadian ACTH rhythm (Szafarczyk et al. 1980a).

Several hypothalamic nuclei send projections to the region of the PVN; among these, the suprachiasmatic nucleus (SCN) stands out as a stimulator of the HPA axis. The SCN has been implicated as a primary regulator of numerous bodily rhythms; accordingly, ablation of the SCN eliminates the circadian corticosterone and ACTH rhythm, blocking the P.M. corticosterone rise (Cascio et al. 1987; Moore and Eichler 1972; Szafarczyk et al. 1979). Unlike input from the brainstem, SCN activation appears to be related to regulation of basal HPA tone rather than communication of information related to stressors.

Selected limbic forebrain areas appear to have excitatory effects on HPA function. Lesion of the central amygdaloid nuclei impairs release of ACTH in response to ether stress, possibly via interactions with serotonergic neurotransmission (Beaulieu et al. 1986). Similarly, bilateral amygdala lesions or interruption of amygdalo-hypothalamic connections significantly reduce the magnitude of the ACTH response to neurogenic stress (Allen and Allen 1974) and block adrenalectomy-induced increases in ACTH release (Allen and Allen

1975). Stimulation of selected sites in the frontal cortex, hippocampus (CA1), amygdala (medial, basomedial, and posteromedial cortical subnuclei), and bed nucleus of the stria terminalis (medial) can elicit release of corticosterone in anesthetized rats (Dunn 1987; Dunn and Orr 1984; Dunn and Whitener 1986; Feldman 1985; Feldman and Conforti 1985), and stimulation of the frontal cortex or preoptic area can excite median-eminence-projecting PVN neurons (Saphier and Feldman 1985).

Stimulatory input into the HPA axis by limbic structures represents an important avenue whereby sensory information can be "shuttled" down to PVN CRH neurons, allowing extraorganismic stimuli to initiate and interact with the HPA response. Interestingly, many studies of limbic excitation of the HPA axis demonstrate considerable response heterogeneity, with responses depending on either the nature of the stressor (Allen and Allen 1974, 1975) or the integrity of various pathways to the PVN (Feldman and Conforti 1985). The data suggest that numerous neuronal circuits may be involved in stimulation of the HPA axis by stimuli from different sensory modalities.

Pathways Involved in Inhibition of the HPA Axis

Inhibition of the HPA axis occurs at two levels—maintaining basal tone of the axis across the circadian period and returning the tone of the axis to the baseline after stimulation (Figure 1-3). Given the potentially deleterious effects of glucocorticoid hypersecretion and the implied connections between HPA disruption and human depressive illness, it is clear that the ability to yoke activation of the axis is as important as the ability to initiate the cascade leading to glucocorticoid release. It is generally agreed that glucocorticoids are responsible for holding HPA activation in check via interactions with brain and/or pituitary glucocorticoid receptors. An extensive literature implicates limbic forebrain structures, including the hippocampus, septum, and possibly amygdala, as putative sites for the hypothesized glucocorticoid negative regulation of HPA function.

One of the ongoing research efforts in our laboratory has been the study of hippocampal pathways governing regulation of the CRH neuron (Table 1-1). We have demonstrated a distinct inhibitory effect of the hippocampal formation on basal CRH mRNA synthesis in the rat (Herman et al. 1989a). The inhibitory effect appears to be independent of the direct hippocampal-hypothalamic pathway (the medial corticohypothalamic tract), operating instead via hippocampal efferents in the fornix (Herman et al. 1989b). Because no direct connection exists between the fornix and PVN, it is likely that hippocampal influences on the PVN are relayed through one or more intervening synapses. Potential loci for these synapses include the lateral septum and bed nucleus of the stria terminalis, which receive fibers from CA1-3 and ventral subiculum, respectively (Swanson et al. 1987). As would be expected, tonic inhibition of CRH mRNA synthesis in PVN is accompanied by hippocampal inhibition of basal ACTH and corticosterone secretion. Hippocampectomy, dorsal hippocampectomy, and/or fornix section elicit basal hypersecretion of ACTH and corticosterone (Azmitia and Conrad 1976; Fendler et al. 1961; Fischette et al. 1980; Knigge 1961; Magariños et al. 1987; Moberg et al. 1971; Wilson et al. 1980), whereas hippocampal stimulation (of subfields CA3 and CA4, ventral subiculum, and dentate gyrus) can decrease corticosterone secretion (Dunn and Orr 1984). Electrophysiological data suggest that dorsal hippocampal neurons inhibit median-eminence-projecting PVN neurons (Saphier and Feldman 1987), indicating that actions of hippocampus are registered in appropriate PVN neuronal subpopulations.

In addition to hippocampus, other limbic structures may provide inhibitory input into the HPA sphere of influence. Notably, the lateral septal nuclei have been reported to exert negative regulatory effects on basal HPA function. Basal corticosterone levels are significantly

Table 1-1. Effects of hippocampal lesions on paraventricular nucleus secretagogue mRNA levels

Treatment	Corticotropin-releasing hormone mRNA (fold change)	Arginine vasopressin mRNA (fold change)
Hippocampectomy	3–4	NC
Fornix lesion	2	NC
Medial corticohypothalamic tract lesion	NC	NC
Chronic stress	40%	NC
Adrenalectomy	2–3	8

Note. Data summarize significant changes between control rats and rats with lesions of the hippocampal system. Corticotropin-releasing hormone (CRH) and arginine vasopressin (AVP) mRNA were quantitated in the parvocellular paraventricular nucleus by in situ hybridization histochemistry/autoradiographic image analysis. Included for comparison are results from stressed (7 days of electroconvulsive shock treatment) and adrenalectomized rats. Hippocampectomy and fornix lesion produce changes in CRH mRNA similar in magnitude to adrenalectomy, without markedly affecting AVP mRNA. Medial corticohypothalamic tract lesions, however, are without effect. NC, no significant change.

augmented by lateral septal lesions (Dobrakovova et al. 1982; Nyakas et al. 1979; Usher et al. 1974). Preliminary data from our laboratory indicate that, like hippocampal lesions, mechanical damage to the septum can up-regulate CRH mRNA in PVN (J.P. Herman and S.J. Watson, 1990, unpublished observations). Inhibitory effects of the septum on HPA function are interesting in light of the potential for this region to serve as a relay between hippocampus and PVN; however, the lack of a major projection from lateral septum directly to medial parvocellular PVN neurons (Oldfield and Silverman 1985; Sawchenko and Swanson 1983) indicates that lateral septal interactions require an intervening (presumably hypothalamic) synapse. In addition, stimulation of lateral subdivisions of the bed nucleus of the stria terminalis appears to inhibit corticosterone secretion in anesthetized rats. This region is particularly interesting in hippocampal-HPA interactions, because it provides a potential bisynaptic intercommunication between the ventral hippocampus (and subiculum) and CRH neurons in the PVN (Swanson and Sawchenko 1983; Swanson et al. 1987).

Among hypothalamic nuclei, the ventromedial and arcuate nuclei project to the PVN and have apparent inhibitory effects on HPA function. Ventromedial nucleus lesions increase basal ACTH and corticosterone release (King et al. 1988). Neonatal arcuate nucleus lesions via monosodium glutamate administration also increase A.M. ACTH and corticosterone levels while decreasing corticosterone responses to ether exposure (Dolnikoff et al. 1988). Both manipulations clearly affect metabolism and other endocrine functions, however, somewhat confounding the interpretation of these experiments. Interestingly, our lesion data seem to preclude an influence of direct hippocampal connections to the ventromedial-arcuate on basal HPA tone, in that medial corticohypothalamic tract lesions are ineffective in producing a rise in the PVN CRH message (Herman et al. 1989b). The influence of hypothalamic nuclei providing rich levels of anatomical interaction between the PVN and limbic structures, such as the preoptic nuclei and lateral hypothalamus, remains to be definitively studied.

Inhibition of a stimulated HPA axis can also occur via limbic neurons. Hippocampal ablation can effectively prolong corticosterone responses to restraint stress without affecting the absolute magnitude of the stress response, indicating a role for hippocampal neurons in termination of the stress response (Sapolsky et al. 1984). Lateral septal lesions have been shown to increase the absolute magnitude of the stress response to ether (Seggie et al. 1974). Interestingly, septal ablation can also potentiate the duration of the corticosterone response to immobilization (Dobrakovova et al. 1982), again suggesting some commonality between the septum and hippocampus in HPA regulation.

Glucocorticoid Negative Feedback and the Brain

In recent years, considerable effort has been put forth toward elucidating the brain regions and circuitry responsible for glucocorticoid negative feedback of HPA activation. The presence within the hippocampus of both type I and type II glucocorticoid receptors (Reul and DeKloet 1987), in combination with data suggesting an inhibitory role for the hippocampus in both basal and stimulated HPA activation, clearly implicates the hippocampus as a potential site for negative regulation of the HPA axis by glucocorticoids. However, the presence of type II receptors directly on parvocellular PVN neurons (Fuxe et al. 1985) suggests that blood-borne glucocorticoids may act on this site as well as, or in deference to, the hippocampus to affect HPA function.

Recent data strongly suggest that glucocorticoids may act directly at the level of the PVN to inhibit CRH biosynthesis. Implants of the (type II) glucocorticoid receptor agonist dexamethasone locally in the region of the PVN markedly reduce the up-regulation of CRH mRNA and peptide after opening of the HPA loop by adrenalectomy (Kovacs et al. 1986; Sawchenko 1987a). Conversely, local injection of the type II antagonist RU38486 into the PVN (but not dentate gyrus) provokes an adrenocortical response (DeKloet et al. 1988). Large doses of dexamethasone given systematically to normal rats down-regulate CRH mRNA synthesis in the parvocellular PVN (Kovacs and Mezey 1987; Schäfer et al. 1987). In addition, electrophysiological evidence suggests that glucocorticoids directly inhibit the electrical activity of medial parvocellular PVN neurons (Saphier and Feldman 1988). However, recent data from our laboratory suggest that local PVN receptors may not represent the sole source of glucocorticoid regulation of the CRH neuron (Table 1-2). In an effort to differentiate the effects of neuronal and blood-borne feedback on the CRH neuron, we performed complete deafferentations of the PVN region. Since the vasculature of the PVN remains intact in this lesion, glucocorticoids are in a position to exert feedback effects via the PVN but not via distant structures. Our data indicate that CRH mRNA is markedly increased following deafferentation, to a degree qualitatively similar to that following adrenalectomy (Schäfer et al. 1987; Young et al. 1986) or hippocampal lesion (Herman et al. 1989a). On the other hand, AVP mRNA is not affected to a degree comparable to that seen following adrenalectomy. The results suggest that local

Table 1-2. Effects of hypothalamic deafferentations on HPA function

Treatment	Corticotropin-releasing hormone mRNA (fold change)	Arginine vasopressin mRNA (fold change)	Plasma ACTH	Plasma B
Anterior cut	2–3	2	NC	NC
Posterior cut	NC	NC	Decreased	Decreased
Total cut	2–3	2	Decreased	Decreased
Septal lesion	3	2	NC	NC
Adrenalectomy	2–3	8	Increased	0

Note. Data summarize significant changes between control rats and rats with various hypothalamic deafferentations. Corticotropin-releasing hormone (CRH) and arginine vasopressin (AVP) mRNA were quantitated in the parvocellular paraventricular nucleus by in situ hybridization histochemistry/autoradiographic image analysis. Included for comparison are septal-lesion and adrenalectomized animals. Plasma ACTH and corticosterone (B) were determined in rats subjected to pentobarbital anesthesia and thoracotomy (in preparation for perfusion). Anterior and total cuts yielded increases in CRH mRNA similar to those in adrenalectomized animals, with limited, yet significant, changes in AVP message. Posterior and total cuts yielded lower ACTH and B values than in control animals under the same circumstances (anesthesia and thoracotomy). B levels were above normal in all groups except posterior and total (averages 7–8 μg/dl), reflecting stress associated with perfusion preparation. NC, no significant change.

steroid feedback via PVN type II receptors is not sufficient to maintain normal levels of CRH mRNA expression and, therefore, that neuronal input (perhaps operating via distant glucocorticoid receptors) is actively involved in the maintenance of the basal tone of the CRH neuron (Herman et al. 1990).

In this light, it is important to note that numerous reports support the notion that limbic forebrain structures (in particular, the hippocampal formation) may play a prominent role in steroid-feedback regulation of the HPA axis. There is a body of data indicating that hippocampal damage blocks the ability of dexamethasone to suppress corticosterone secretion in response to stress (Feldman and Conforti 1980; Magariños et al. 1987). Local implants of corticosterone (but not dexamethasone) into the dorsal hippocampus can reverse the up-regulation of CRH peptide expression (Kovacs et al. 1986) and the hypersecretion of ACTH (Kovacs and Makara 1988) seen following adrenalectomy. Furthermore, an elegant series of studies by Sapolsky et al. (1986) draws remarkable (inverse) correlations between the hippocampal glucocorticoid receptor number and the ability to terminate the adrenocortical stress response in pathological and aged states.

An explanation for glucocorticoid regulation of the HPA axis by local PVN type II receptors and distant limbic receptors may lie in the necessity for multiple levels of steroid regulation of the HPA axis. For instance, it is clear that appropriate termination of the stress response is as vital to survival as its initiation, in that excessive secretion of glucocorticoids has multiple deleterious effects on the organism. Therefore, it would make sense for glucocorticoids to have access to secretory (i.e., PVN) neurons and maintain an ability to shut down ACTH secretagogues after stressful episodes. For regulation of basal HPA fluctuations, however, a more subtle regulation is required. It is evident that the SCN is a prime mover of P.M. adrenocortical activation in the rat. The mechanisms establishing circadian shutdown are, however, unclear. Interestingly, one of the consistent findings after hippocampal damage or fornix lesion is a desynchronization of the circadian corticosterone (and ACTH) rhythm (Azmitia and Conrad 1976; Fischette et al. 1980; Moberg et al. 1971; Wilson et al. 1980). Hippocampal damage apparently yokes the tone of the HPA axis to a constant level, with corticosterone values holding between A.M. and P.M. values. Binding studies suggest that hippocampal type I receptors, in particular, seem to be in a position to support influences on circadian HPA function. Dallman et al. (1987) reported that the hippocampal type I receptors appear to be extensively occupied at levels of circulating free corticosterone found throughout most of the circadian cycle. Circadian activation of the HPA axis coincides well with those points in time when free type I receptors can be observed (Dallman et al. 1989), suggesting an inverse relationship between activation and type I binding. Type I (but not type II) binding in the hippocampus also shows A.M.-P.M. variation (Reul and DeKloet 1987), suggesting a circadian rhythmicity of receptor synthesis. These data, in combination with our results demonstrating up-regulation of CRH mRNA levels after A.M. hippocampal ablation, provide a basis for a role for hippocampal type I receptors in circadian *inhibition* of HPA function and hence a mechanism whereby glucocorticoids can establish the tone of neuroendocrine systems governing their release.

PITUITARY STEROID FEEDBACK

In addition to multiple sites in the brain, a pituitary site of action for glucocorticoids is clear. Thus, it can be demonstrated that glucocorticoids have direct effects on POMC gene transcription, mRNA levels, and subsequent peptide stores in vitro in primary pituitary cultures (Birnberg et al. 1983; Roberts et al. 1979a; Schacter et al. 1982). These pituitary effects appear to act through the classic glucocorticoid receptor (type II), which binds glucocorticoids, is translocated to the nucleus, and binds to sites on the DNA (Sakly and Koch 1981). In the case of POMC, this binding site should turn off transcription of the POMC gene (Schacter et al. 1982). This transcriptional regulation affects pituitary stores of ACTH and related peptides. These genomic effects are the best understood of the negative feedback effects of glucocorticoids. Studies by several groups have demonstrated that glucocorticoids may interact with the CRH receptor in the anterior pituitary, acutely inhibiting the binding of CRH to its receptor and chronically decreasing the CRH receptor number (Childs et al. 1986; Schwartz et al. 1986). Such direct effects of glucocorticoids on CRH receptors may account for some of the inhibitory action of glucocorticoids on ACTH release in vitro; however, the importance of CNS circuitry versus the pituitary as the primary regulatory site is still being explored. Our studies demonstrate a direct inhibitory effect of glucocorticoids on corticotroph secretion in vitro (Figure 1-4). This is a modest effect, and glucocorticoids inhibit CRH-stimulated release by 50% at best. Glucocorticoids do not inhibit basal release. In contrast, the inhibitory effects of glucocorticoids in vivo (Figure 1-5) appear to be more profound, suggesting that in vivo glucocorticoids act at both central and pituitary sites.

Dallman et al. (1987) also addressed the issue of pituitary versus brain glucocorticoid feedback in vivo. With the use of ADX rats that

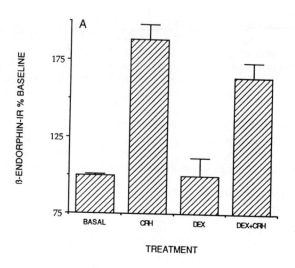

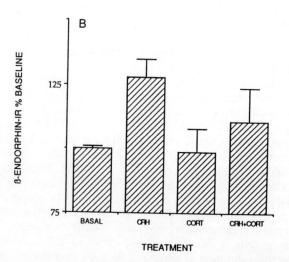

Figure 1-4. Effect of glucocorticoids in vitro on corticotropin-releasing hormone (CRH)–stimulated release of β-endorphin from anterior lobe corticotrophs. In both cases, CRH stimulated release of β-endorphin, and dexamethasone (DEX, *A*) and corticosterone (CORT, *B*) were able to antagonize partially this CRH-stimulated release when administered concomitantly with CRH for 60 minutes. These data support direct effect of glucocorticoids at pituitary in a short time frame.

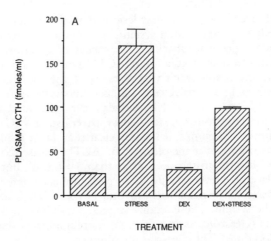

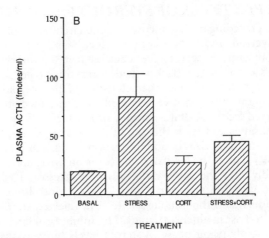

Figure 1-5. Effects of glucocorticoids in vivo on stress-induced ACTH release. *A*: Dexamethasone (DEX) was administered 90 minutes before administration of 30 minutes of intermittent foot-shock stress. *B*: Corticosterone (CORT) was administered immediately before administration of 5 minutes of swim stress. In both feedback paradigms, glucocorticoids inhibited corticotroph's response to stress but had no effect on non–stress-driven plasma ACTH levels. Effect of glucocorticoids in vivo appears greater than effect in vitro (see Figure 1-4), suggesting that glucocorticoids turn off corticotropin-releasing hormone secretion and block ACTH release from pituitary.

had received hypothalamic lesions that disconnected the PVN from the hypophyseal portal system, they demonstrated that removal of glucocorticoid feedback in the absence of CRH drive had no effect on the pituitary regulation of ACTH synthesis and secretion. In this case, the brain circuitry appears to be the most important site of feedback in adrenalectomy-induced hypersecretion of ACTH. In a related experiment with hypothalamic lesioned rats and graded doses of corticosterone replacement with constant CRH infusion with osmotic minipumps, it became clear that direct inhibitory effects of corticosteroids at the pituitary on ACTH release require concentrations of corticosterone greater than 10 µg/dl, but corticosterone replacement levels of 5 µg/dl turn off adrenalectomy-induced ACTH hypersecretion in animals with intact hypothalamo-pituitary elements of the system. These studies suggest that glucocorticoid control of CRH release via brain circuitry is more important than its inhibitory action on ACTH release at the pituitary.

MULTIPLE TYPES OF STEROID FEEDBACK

The preceding review focuses on the circuitry involved in HPA axis activation and glucocorticoid feedback. From a physiological standpoint, however, feedback is not a unitary phenomenon. Glucocorticoid feedback is divided into three types of feedback based on time domains and characteristics of the steroid-administration paradigm: rate-sensitive fast feedback, intermediate feedback, and delayed feedback. Rate-sensitive or fast feedback is active in seconds to minutes and reads the rate of rise of steroids in plasma following stress-induced rises or administration of steroids (Dallman and Yates 1969). This is the feedback that turns off CRH and ACTH secretion rapidly after the application of a brief stressor. Dallman and Yates (1969), Hillhouse and Jones (1976), and Jones et al. (1972) demonstrated the inhibitory effects of injected steroids on a stress-induced rise in glucocorticoids. This inhibitory effect occurred during the rapidly rising phase of steroid levels but was absent during the plateau phase of steroid levels, even when high levels were present. Rate-sensitive feedback can be demonstrated even when already-high levels of steroids are present in plasma, as long as there is a rising steroid level. Beginning 30–90 minutes after steroid administration, intermediate, level-sensitive feedback proportional to the total dose of steroids administered is demonstrable. Rate-sensitive and proportional feedback inhibit CRH-driven ACTH secretion; neither of these affects the basal level of ACTH secretion in vivo or in vitro in anterior pituitary explants or primary cultures (Dallman et al. 1987; Jones et al. 1974). In contrast, slow or delayed feedback occurs at the genomic level and therefore decreases pituitary stores, thus affecting both basal and CRH-driven ACTH secretion (Roberts et al. 1979a, 1979b). Although these types of feedback are clearly demonstrable in vivo and, in some cases, in vitro, the association of these types of feedback with the sites of feedback and the cellular mechanisms underlying these types of controls is unclear. Similarly, the interaction of these various feedback sites in a hierarchical fashion is also unclear. Older studies suggested that fast feedback occurred primarily in brain, although inhibitory effects of corticosterone in vitro at the pituitary can be demonstrated in 15 minutes (Dallman et al. 1987; Widmaier and Dallman 1983). Inhibitory effects of an injected steroid on a subsequent in vitro pituitary response to secretagogues have also been well known for several years. These data suggest a pituitary site for intermediate feedback; however, in vitro studies can never directly identify the primary sites of steroid feedback, because only one level of the HPA axis can be addressed.

NEW APPROACHES TO THE HPA AXIS

Given that the HPA axis is a closed-loop system with nested feedback loops, what are the likely areas to target in HPA axis studies of depression? There are no truly satisfactory animal models of depression. Nevertheless, chronic stress is a paradigm that helps us to understand HPA regulation at multiple levels (molecular, cellular, and system). This is not to suggest that stress and depression are equivalent, but the compensatory brain and pituitary mechanisms of HPA oversecretion have been well studied in rodents and can be useful in addressing the neuroendocrine changes in depression. Using chronic intermittent foot shock as a model system, we have characterized numerous changes that occur with chronic stress. Initial studies focused on the anterior pituitary corticotroph.

Basic Studies

Thirty minutes of intermittent foot shock is accompanied by release of ACTH into plasma and a decrease in corticotroph content of ACTH to approximately 75% of control (Young and Akil 1985). When this same stressor is repeated for 14 days and the animals are sacrificed 24 hours after the last stress session (chronic stress/rest), there is an increase in corticotroph ACTH content to 200% of control. This increase occurs despite continued release of similar amounts of ACTH into plasma with repeated foot-shock stress (Figure 1-6). Consequently, in this case an increased content of the corticotroph occurs not because of diminished release but because of the facilitatory influences of chronic stress on the anterior pituitary corticotroph. This

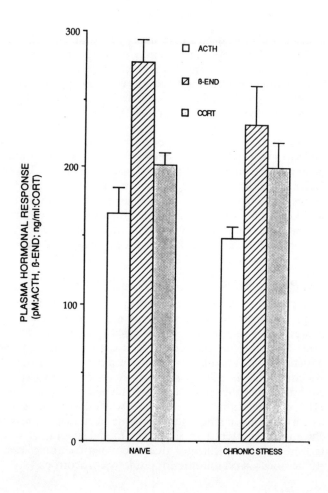

Figure 1-6. ACTH, β-endorphin (β-END), and corticosterone (CORT) response to 1st and 15th foot-shock stress sessions in rats. This stressor resulted in release of ACTH, β-endorphin, and corticosterone in both stress sessions, with little difference between sessions because various adaptations in hypothalamic-pituitary-adrenal axis acted to maintain same response for repeated stress.

increased content occurs despite the high levels of glucocorticoids secreted in response to foot-shock stress. This suggests that the feed-forward elements of the system (CRH, AVP) are stronger than the feedback elements (glucocorticoids) and that POMC biosynthesis is relatively insensitive to negative feedback in situations of chronic demand. When rats are restressed before sacrifice, there is a substantial release of ACTH into plasma as well as a decrease in corticotroph ACTH content relative to the chronic stress/rest baseline. The content is still elevated compared with control rats, but the magnitude of the increase is much smaller than the increase in chronically stressed/rested rats. In this case, pituitary ACTH and β-endorphin content data could be misleading, because the small changes in ACTH content demonstrable after chronic or acute stress could easily be missed. In these situations, POMC mRNA levels in the pituitary can provide valuable additional information critical to confirming the chronically increased drive to the corticotroph. Because mRNA levels integrate during a longer time frame (hours to days), this measure is relatively insensitive to acute changes but accurately reflects chronic drive. In the case of foot-shock stress, POMC mRNA levels are unchanged after acute stress but elevated after chronic stress (Shiomi et al. 1986). This acute stressor severely depletes the ACTH content of the pituitary (75% of control), so a mechanism for rapidly replenishing the ACTH stores is necessary. In situations of chronic demand, however, the system depends on the increased protein stores and increased mRNA levels to meet the demands of repeated stress.

How do these various adaptations in the corticotroph affect response to CRH? To answer this question, we directly examined the pituitary's response to AVP and CRH in vitro in three stress conditions (acute, chronic/rest, and chronic/acute) and in control rats (Young and Akil 1985). Acute foot-shock stress is accompanied by a diminished ACTH and β-endorphin response of the corticotroph to AVP and CRH in vitro. This is not so with chronic stress. Pituitaries from the chronic/acute stress rats demonstrated an increased response to CRH. Consequently, the same challenge (acute foot-shock stress) leads to a decreased response to CRH in the pituitary from a naive rat and an increased response to CRH in the pituitary after repeated challenge. The increased release of ACTH and β-endorphin with CRH in the chronic/acute stress group again suggested a facilitatory influence of increased drive on responsiveness to CRH. It also suggests a possible insensitivity to negative feedback at the pituitary. This hypothesis was tested directly by adding glucocorticoids in vitro to anterior pituitary preparations from control and chronically stressed rats. In control-rat pituitaries, both corticosterone and dexamethasone caused a 50% decrease in CRH-stimulated release of β-endorphin. Neither steroid affected basal (unstimulated) release. In pituitaries from chronically stressed rats, this inhibition of CRH-driven release was absent. In fact, both corticosterone and dexamethasone caused a 50% increase in β-endorphin release over CRH, suggesting a switch from negative to positive feedback at the pituitary (Young and Akil 1988). Again, all of these changes are observable at one level of the HPA axis, the pituitary corticotroph. Other changes may occur at higher levels, such as the brain.

To explore adaptation at the hypothalamic level of the HPA axis, another stressor, electroconvulsive seizure (ECS), was used in a chronic-stress paradigm. Like chronic foot-shock stress, chronic ECS leads to an increase in pituitary ACTH content and an increase in POMC mRNA in the pituitary. In the brain, chronic ECS leads to increased CRH mRNA but a decreased CRH content in the parvocellular neurons of the PVN. In this case, mRNA levels were able to demonstrate an increased drive for secretion when peptide-content levels of CRH were actually decreased (Herman et al. 1989c). Again, these data suggest the importance of measures that integrate for longer time frames than peptide content, which is subject to acute release with consequent decreases in content.

These studies demonstrate some of the changes that occur at multiple levels of the HPA axis with chronic stress. But how are these changes integrated in vivo? Are there changes in HPA axis regulation in vivo after chronic stress? The answer is different depending on the various challenges used to probe the system. In some cases regulation can appear completely normal. The response to the 1st and 15th foot-shock stress session is one example (Figure 1-6). In this case, the ACTH, β-endorphin, and corticosterone responses to foot-shock stress are almost identical in naive and chronically stressed rats. Adaptations at various levels of the HPA axis act to maintain the proper level of response (ACTH and corticosterone) to foot-shock stress. If these chronically stressed rats receive a different stressor, however, 5 minutes of swim stress (Figure 1-7), a much greater response to stress is seen. These data demonstrate that the response of the HPA axis may depend on the familiarity as well as the magnitude of the stressor.

To examine glucocorticoid feedback in vivo, a fast-feedback model was chosen because 1) fast feedback affects ACTH release in vivo and 2) fast feedback appears to act at the brain to turn off CRH release rather than acting at the pituitary, as is the case with longer-term feedback. A fast-feedback paradigm was developed in conjunction with Mary Dallman (Young et al. 1990a). The same chronic-stress

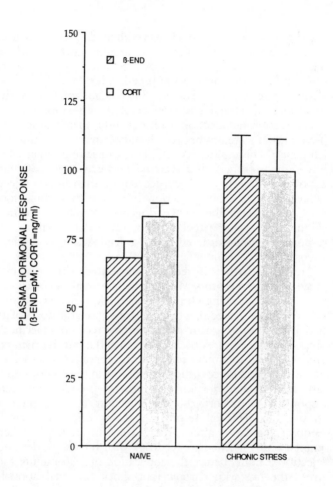

Figure 1-7. β-endorphin (β-END) and corticosterone (CORT) response to 5-minute 25° centigrade swim session involving naive rats and rats that received chronic foot shock for 14 days. Rats that were chronically stressed demonstrated an increased response to this novel stressor compared with naive rats. Similarly, there was increased corticosterone secretion after 5 minutes. These data contrast with data from Figure 1-6, demonstrating the same response to a repeated stressor, foot-shock stress, and highlight that different probes (foot-shock vs. swim stress) can produce different pictures of hypothalamic-pituitary-adrenal axis regulation in vivo.

paradigm, chronic foot shock, was evaluated for changes in sensitivity to fast feedback. Injection of corticosterone (instead of saline) immediately before the application of a brief stressor (5-minute swim) resulted in a rapid decrease in β-endorphin (and ACTH) secretion after the stressor in a naive rat. This was not so in rats with chronic foot shock, who failed to turn off secretion of β-endorphin in response to corticosterone injection. Consequently, there was no decrease in β-endorphin secretion between 5 and 30 minutes (Figure 1-8, lower left panel). This diminished ACTH response resulted in substantially less corticosterone being secreted between 5 and 30 minutes in control rats injected with corticosterone than in rats injected with saline. Corticosterone injection in rats with chronic foot shock resulted in little inhibition of endogenous secretion of corticosterone (Figure 1-8, upper panel). Again, these data confirm an altered response to glucocorticoid negative feedback in vivo after chronic stress.

Are these changes in feedback associated with changes in brain glucocorticoid receptors? We have no data on glucocorticoid receptor levels in rats receiving chronic foot shock; however, Sapolsky et al. (1986) demonstrated that chronic stress and large doses of glucocorticoids can down-regulate glucocorticoid receptors specifically in the hippocampus. Fast feedback was evaluated in rats receiving the same glucocorticoid treatment regimen that Sapolsky et al. demonstrated down-regulated glucocorticoid receptors in the hippocampus. These rats demonstrated a failure to turn off β-endorphin secretion in response to acute corticosterone injection similar to the chronically stressed rats. This failure provides strong evidence of altered CNS feedback regulation after chronic stress. Interestingly, when we examined only intermediate feedback with the use of dexamethasone injection 2 hours before the application of a 30-minute foot-shock stress, the rats with chronic foot shock appeared normal. Again, these data demonstrate the independence of fast feedback from intermediate-feedback abnormalities, emphasize the importance of multiple probes used to challenge the HPA axis, and emphasize the importance of the brain over the pituitary as a site of feedback control.

Clinical Studies

Most of the earlier studies on HPA axis regulation have focused on dexamethasone as a challenge and examined the 4 P.M. time period the day after dexamethasone administration. This time period was chosen empirically but clearly presents a balance between a possible increased CNS drive in depression and a decreased sensitivity to the negative feedback effects of dexamethasone. These studies appear to

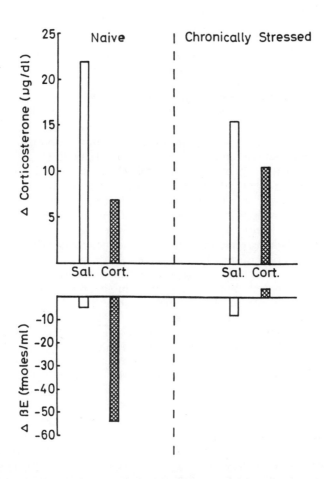

Figure 1-8. Fast-feedback data from rats administered chronic foot shock. In naive rat receiving 5 minutes of swim stress, stress-induced ACTH secretion resulted in a substantial increase in corticosterone secretion between end of stressor and peak corticosterone secretion (30 minutes). When corticosterone was administered before stress, little endogenous corticosterone was secreted in response to stress (upper left panel). This diminished corticosterone secretion was secondary to shutting off corticotroph secretion (β-endorphin [βE], lower left panel). In rats receiving chronic foot shock there was little decrease in endogenous corticosterone secretion after corticosterone injection before stress (compare saline [Sal.] and corticosterone [Cort.], upper right panel). Plasma β-endorphin levels confirm that in chronically stressed rats, the corticotroph does not turn off secretion appropriately after corticosterone injection.

emphasize the intermediate-to-late feedback effects of dexamethasone; the anatomical site of action of dexamethasone is unclear but probably involves pituitary sites instead of brain sites. The use of a cutoff value to define cortisol nonsuppressors favors the classification of those individuals with increased cortisol levels secondary to adrenal hypertrophy as nonsuppressors rather than individuals with faulty feedback only. In addition, most studies have assumed that only the dexamethasone nonsuppressors demonstrate abnormal HPA axis regulation. Our studies on depression indicate this is not always so. In our studies examining β-endorphin levels in plasma before and after dexamethasone administration, many individuals demonstrated a failure to suppress β-endorphin with dexamethasone (Matthews et al. 1986). Previous studies demonstrated that as a group, normal control subjects decreased plasma β-endorphin levels to 48% of their baseline values, whereas endogenously depressed patients suppressed β-endorphin to 63% of their baseline values. With an individual criterion to classify patients as suppressors or nonsuppressors, 50% of the patients demonstrated abnormal β-endorphin suppression with dexamethasone. One-third of the patients demonstrated failure to suppress cortisol, and the two groups did not always overlap. Consequently, by use of the same probe, dexamethasone, but assessing two levels of the HPA axis simultaneously (adrenal and pituitary), abnormal HPA axis regulation in 72% of depressed subjects was demonstrated. We continued to examine the corticotroph's response to dexamethasone in normal control subjects and depressed patients. Figure 1-9 demonstrates the plasma β-endorphin and cortisol response to dexamethasone in a group of 16 control subjects and 31 depressed subjects. Although both groups demonstrate suppression of β-endorphin, this suppression is small in depressed subjects, particularly in contrast to the control subjects. However, both groups demonstrate similar cortisol suppression. Again, this suppression points out that several depressed patients who are dexamethasone suppressors by cortisol criteria still demonstrate abnormal corticotroph regulation in response to dexamethasone challenge. Dexamethasone, as used in this standard fashion, evaluates primarily pituitary feedback, because it is not taken up by the hippocampus, and the time domains of this feedback suggest primary regulation at the pituitary. Consequently, despite the demonstration of clear abnormal corticotroph regulation, it is important to pursue newer approaches. Studies with other challenges may provide further evidence of HPA dysregulation at multiple levels of the HPA axis.

Several groups have published studies on the response to CRH in depressed and control subjects. All groups agree that depression

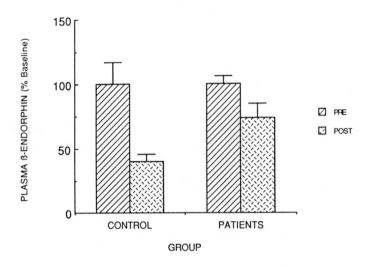

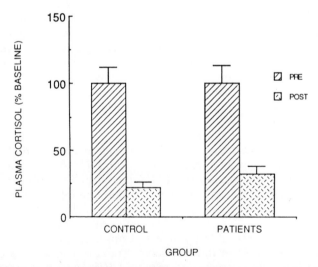

Figure 1-9. Corticotroph and adrenal response to dexamethasone in control and depressed subjects. The day after dexamethasone administration at 11:30 P.M., control subjects demonstrated suppression of plasma β-endorphin levels to 45% of their baseline at 4 P.M. In contrast, depressed patients only suppressed plasma β-endorphin to 75% of their baseline. Both groups demonstrated clear suppression of plasma cortisol. PRE, before dexamethasone administration; POST, after dexamethasone administration.

results in a decreased corticotroph response to CRH, but the interpretation of this finding is subject to debate (Amsterdam et al. 1987;
Gold et al. 1986; Holsboer et al. 1984; Young et al. 1990b). Most
of the studies have identified the hypercortisolism of depression as
contributing to the diminished ACTH response to CRH (Gold et al.
1986; Holsboer et al. 1984); however, our studies (Young et al.
1990b) and those of Amsterdam et al. (1987) demonstrated abnormal responses to CRH in patients without demonstrable hypercortisolemia. In our studies, we divided patients by baseline cortisol into
three groups (high, low, and normal baseline cortisol) and observed
nearly identical, decreased integrated β-endorphin responses (area
under the curve) in all three groups (Figure 1-10), suggesting that
baseline cortisol levels were not the critical variable in explaining the
decreased corticotroph response to CRH. Our data and those of
Amsterdam et al. (1987) also demonstrated a normal initial secretory
response (Δ-β-endorphin or Δ-ACTH) despite a markedly decreased
integrated corticotroph response. However, the cortisol response
varied by resting cortisol values: Subjects with either high or low
baseline cortisol response demonstrated integrated cortisol responses
smaller than those of normal subjects; subjects with resting cortisol
values in the normal range demonstrated integrated cortisol responses
identical to those of normal control subjects (Figure 1-10). Interestingly, the individuals with high resting cortisol demonstrated cortisol
secretory activity during the hour preceding the CRH infusion. We
believe that this activity may be a nonspecific stress response to the
first placebo injection, but we can not exclude spontaneous secretory
activity.

Does this pre-CRH secretory activity affect the response to CRH?
The work of Rivier and Vale (1983) in rats receiving multiple doses
of CRH demonstrated an acute desensitization to CRH for several
hours after administration of CRH. Although glucocorticoid negative
feedback plays a role in this desensitization, this inhibitory effect was
observed in adrenalectomized rats, pointing to direct effects on CRH
receptors themselves, perhaps because of some acute change in the
coupling to second messengers. Consequently, the decreased
response to CRH in those patients demonstrating active secretion
may be caused by desensitization of the CRH receptor after secretion
of endogenous CRH. Again, these data point to a more complicated
alteration in depressed patients than just intermediate steroid feedback inhibiting the responsiveness to CRH. Since all of these studies
in humans were conducted with endogenous CRH and AVP secretion, changes in the endogenous secretion of these hormones may
alter responsiveness to exogenous CRH. Similarly, it is possible that

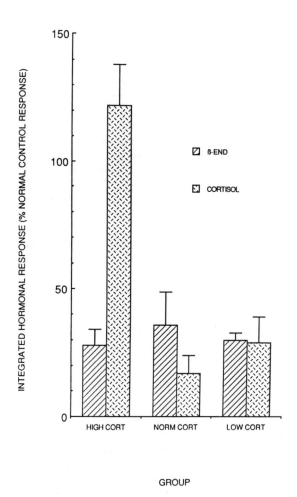

Figure 1-10. Comparison of integrated β-endorphin (β-END) response and integrated cortisol response in depressed patients divided into three groups by their cortisol (CORT) levels before receiving corticotropin-releasing hormone (CRH). All groups demonstrated remarkably decreased integrated β-endorphin response to CRH (approximately 30% of control). Patients with high and low resting cortisols also demonstrated decreased integrated cortisol response to CRH. Patients with normal (NORM) resting cortisol levels, however, demonstrated normal to increased cortisol response to CRH, even though these same patients demonstrated profoundly decreased corticotroph response to CRH.

cortisol secreted in response to CRH feeds back to affect the corticotroph's response to exogenous CRH in the later phase of the CRH response. Decreases in the number of CRH receptors on the pituitary cannot be excluded (Nemeroff et al. 1984). Consequently, a question remains: How do we find probes that bring us closer to the brain? Steroid feedback may again provide some clues.

As described in the basic science review, glucocorticoid fast feedback operates for short time frames and appears to involve brain circuits to turn off CRH secretion. In humans, fast feedback can be studied by infusion of cortisol at times of high circadian CRH drive (morning). We have begun fast-feedback studies in humans and are able to demonstrate a clear effect of cortisol infusion on β-endorphin secretion in normal control subjects. Studies on depressed subjects are now in progress and suggest that there are abnormalities in this form of feedback in depressed subjects. Such a finding can lead us one step closer to the brain. Other areas that remain to be explored in vivo are the role of glucocorticoid receptor heterogeneity in controlling HPA axis abnormalities and the reevaluation of evidence for increased circadian drive in the evening. The increasing availability of specific glucocorticoid agonists and antagonists offers new probes for future in vivo studies. The new techniques of molecular biology combined with postmortem tissues can provide new clues to pituitary and brain regulation in depression.

Postmortem/Molecular Biology Approach

Recent technological breakthroughs in neuroscience have made possible the direct study of HPA axis structures in human tissue. Even though autopsy material has some intrinsic problems, such as the effect of postmortem delay on molecular and cellular processes, its advantage is that it puts us into a position whereby we can study the tissue itself. Preliminary rat studies in our laboratories suggest that in the pituitary, no POMC mRNA loss or degradation is detected in the first 24 hours after death, but more studies are needed to clarify the effect of postmortem time on different mRNA species in different tissues. By applying the same experimental approach that has been used in animal studies, we can begin to ask questions about the neuroendocrine stress circuit in humans and interpret the results in light of what we know about the regulation of this system in laboratory animals. For example, measurement of mRNA content in specific brain regions can give us an idea of the overall tone of the system. Since we have learned from animal studies that, at least in some tissues, changes in the total mRNA pool do not occur with a single secretory episode (Shiomi et al. 1986), measuring message levels of specific stress-related peptides, such as POMC and CRH, may give us an idea of the history of the system before death. If we combine mRNA quantification with peptide measurement by radioimmunoassay and receptor binding in the same or parallel tissues, we can begin to understand how different cellular components of the system are related. Furthermore, if we extend this cellular analysis to the different tissues that form part of the HPA axis, we will be able to obtain a more complete neurochemical profile of the stress axis and the biochemical events that underlie regulation of the different levels of the system.

Although there have been several postmortem studies of the classical neurotransmitter systems in brains of psychiatric patients (mostly receptor binding and content), less attention has been paid to the components of the HPA axis. Nemeroff et al. (1984) found decreased ovine CRH receptor binding in the frontal cortex of suicide victims. Even though this observation suggests increased activity of the cortical CRH system, it does not necessarily follow that there is increased CRH secretion from the PVN into the portal circulation. Dorovini-Zis and Zis (1987) showed increased adrenal weight in suicide victims, again providing more evidence suggesting chronic CRH and ACTH hypersecretion in depression.

We have approached the postmortem study of the human HPA axis by using in situ hybridization. This is a histochemical technique in which endogenous mRNA is detected in tissue sections via a radioactive nucleic acid complementary to the molecule of interest. It allows quantification of different mRNA species in a precise neuroanatomical context by using different probes in adjacent sections (Watson et al. 1987). It also allows for the use of receptor autoradiography in the same area so that the relationship between receptor and mRNA regulation can be studied. When in situ hybridization is combined with cellular stains, such as thionin or hematoxylin eosin, the resolution of this technique allows us to quantify the amount of mRNA per cell. This is helpful in determining whether changes in tissue mRNA are caused by changes in total cell number (e.g., hyperplasia) or increases in mRNA copies per cell.

We showed the feasibility of this approach in a pilot study (López et al. 1988) that used pituitaries of suicide and cardiac-death victims for adjacent-section in situ hybridization and receptor autoradiography. We were able to visualize the close anatomical association between cells containing POMC mRNA (corticotrophs) and CRH receptors in human anterior pituitaries. In addition, we observed that glucocorticoid receptor mRNA is present not only in corticotrophs containing POMC but in other pituitary cells as well. This level of resolution allows us to address specific regulatory issues, such as 1) the relationship between changes in receptor binding and changes in mRNA content in the same groups of pituitary cells and 2) the regulation of the glucocorticoid receptor mRNA associated with corticotrophs as opposed to the glucocorticoid mRNA associated with noncorticotrophic cells.

With the use of in situ hybridization, we detected a small but significant increase in POMC mRNA in the pituitaries of 7 suicide victims compared to 11 pituitaries of cardiac-death control subjects. When a more detailed analysis was carried out combining in situ hybridization and thionin staining, we were able to ascertain that this increase in POMC mRNA was caused by a higher mRNA content per cell in the corticotrophs of suicide victims. These findings are consistent with the increase in POMC mRNA observed in the pituitaries of chronically stressed rats and are suggestive of CRH hypersecretion.

An alternative method to study regulation is by extracting the tissue of interest and measuring mRNA content by Northern blot or another similar technique. We also measured POMC mRNA by Northern and dot blot techniques and found the same increase in the pituitaries of suicide victims (J. López, M. Arato, S.J. Watson, unpublished observations, 1989). Although mRNA quantification by this method does not allow the visualization of the cells in their anatomical context, it can be used to concomitantly measure peptide content by radioimmunoassay in the same tissue. With this approach, we can study the relationship between transcriptional and translational activity in the different compartments of the HPA axis.

The extension of the strategies of molecular biology to the human brain regions that we discussed previously as part of the HPA circuitry will elucidate how the different HPA elements are regulated in depression. It will perhaps lead us to a better understanding of the regulatory biology of the limbic system with regard to stress and of the relevance of these mechanisms to mental illness.

SUMMARY

Brain circuitry plays a critical role in HPA axis regulation. Because of this role of the brain, the HPA axis is often viewed as a window to the brain. Most studies of depression have focused on corticotroph or adrenal regulation with the use of dexamethasone or CRH as challenges. Although studies focusing on these peripheral hormones can provide clues to the abnormalities of depression, newer strategies for moving closer to the brain are necessary. As basic animal research on the brain circuitry controlling HPA axis regulation progresses, these newer strategies for challenging the HPA axis will develop. The techniques of molecular biology provide critical probes to explore cellular and systemwide regulation in the brain and its periphery in depressed patients. The availability of postmortem brain tissue coupled with molecular biology is one exciting advance in bringing us closer to understanding the multiple changes and adaptations that occur centrally in depression.

REFERENCES

Abou-Samra A-B, Harwood JP, Manganiello VC, et al: Phorbol 12-myristate 13 acetate and vasopressin potentiate the effect of corticotropin-releasing factor on cyclic AMP production in rat anterior pituitary cells: mechanisms of action. J Biol Chem 262:1129–1136, 1987

Affolter HU, Reisine T: Corticotropin releasing factor increases proopiomelanocortin messenger RNA in mouse anterior pituitary tumor cells. J Biol Chem 260:15477–15481, 1985

Aguilera G, Harwood JP, Wilson JX, et al: Mechanism of action of corticotropin releasing factor and other regulators of corticotropin release in rat pituitary cells. J Biol Chem 258:8039–8045, 1983

Akil H, Ueda Y, Lin H-L: A sensitive coupled HPLC/RIA technique for separation of endorphins: multiple forms of β-endorphin in rat pituitary intermediate vs. anterior lobe. Neuropeptide 1:429–446, 1981

Akil H, Shiomi H, Mathews J: Induction of the intermediate pituitary by stress: synthesis and release of a non-opioid form of β-endorphin. Science 227:424–426, 1985

Allen JP, Allen CF: Role of the amygdaloid complexes in the stress-induced release of ACTH in the rat. Neuroendocrinology 15:220–230, 1974

Allen JP, Allen CF: Amygdalar participation in tonic ACTH secretion in the rat. Neuroendocrinology 19:115–125, 1975

Alonso G, Szafarczyk A, Balmefrezol M, et al: Immunocytochemical evidence for stimulatory control by the ventral noradrenergic bundle of parvocellular neurons of the paraventricular nucleus secreting corticotropin releasing hormone and vasopressin in rats. Brain Res 397:297–307, 1986

Amsterdam JC, Winokur A, Abelman E, et al: Co-syntropin (ACTH a^{1-24}) stimulation test in depressed patients and healthy subjects. Am J Psychiatry 140:907–909, 1983

Amsterdam JD, Maislin G, Winokur A, et al: Pituitary and adrenocortical responses to ovine corticotropin releasing hormone in depressed patients and healthy volunteers. Arch Gen Psychiatry 44:775–781, 1987

Antoni FA: Hypothalamic control of adrenocorticotropin secretion: advances since the discovery of 41-residue corticotropin-releasing factor. Endocr Rev 7:351–378, 1986

Antoni FA, Palkovits M, Makara G, et al: Immunoreactive corticotropin-releasing hormone (CRF) in the hypothalamo-infundibular tract. Neuroendocrinology 36:415–432, 1983

Axelrod J, Reisine TD: Stress hormones: their interaction and regulation. Science 224:452–459, 1984

Azmitia EC Jr, Conrad LCA: Temporal effects of fornix transection on brain tryptophan hydroxylase activity and plasma corticosterone levels. Neuroendocrinology 21:338–349, 1976

Baertsch AJ, Friedli M: A novel type of vasopressin receptor on anterior pituitary corticotrophs? Endocrinology 116:499–502, 1985

Beaulieu S, DiPoalo T, Barden N: Control of ACTH secretion by the central nucleus of the amygdala: implication of the serotonergic system and its relevance to the glucocorticoid delayed negative feedback mechanism. Neuroendocrinology 44:247–254, 1986

Beresford TP, Shankar TP, Solomon SS, et al: ACTH levels during cortisol suppression (letter). Am J Psychiatry 142:526, 1985

Berger M, Pirker KM, Krieg CJ, et al: ACTH and cortisol levels in healthy probands and psychiatric patients following the dexamethasone suppression test. Am J Psychiatry 142:268–269, 1985

Bethune JE: The diagnosis and treatment of adrenal insufficiency, in Endocrinology, Vol 2. Edited by DeGroot LJ. Philadelphia, PA, WB Saunders, 1989, pp 1647–1659

Bilezikjian LM, Vale W: Glucocorticoids inhibit CRF induced production of cAMP in cultured anterior pituitary cells. Endocrinology 113:657–662, 1983

Birnberg NC, Lissitsky JC, Hinman M, et al: Glucocorticoids regulate pro-opiomelanocortin gene expression at the level of transcription and secretion. Proc Natl Acad Sci USA 80:6982–6986, 1983

Bruhn TO, Plotsky PM, Vale WW: Effect of paraventricular lesions on corticotropin-releasing factor-like immunoreactivity in the stalk-median eminence: studies on the adrenocorticotropin response to ether stress and CRF. Endocrinology 114:57–62, 1984

Carroll BJ, Curtis GC, Mendels J: Neuroendocrine regulation in depression, I: limbic system adrenocortical dysfunction. Arch Gen Psychiatry 33:1039–1044, 1976a

Carroll BJ, Curtis GC, Mendels J: Neuroendocrine regulation in depression,

II: discrimination of depressed from non-depressed subjects. Arch Gen Psychiatry 33:1051–1058, 1976b

Carroll BJ, Feinberg M, Greden JF, et al: A specific laboratory test for the diagnosis of melancholia: standardization, validation and clinical utility. Arch Gen Psychiatry 38:15–22, 1981

Cascio CS, Shinsako J, Dallman MF: The suprachiasmatic nuclei stimulate evening ACTH secretion in the rat. Brain Res 423:173–178, 1987

Childs GV, Morell JL, Niendorf A, et al: Cytochemical studies of corticotropin releasing factor receptors in anterior lobe corticotrophs: binding, glucocorticoid regulation and endocytosis of [Biotinyl-Ser[1]] CRF. Endocrinology 119:2129–2142, 1986

Cohen MR, Pickar D, Extein I, et al: Plasma cortisol and β-endorphin immunoreactivity in nonmajor and major depression. Am J Psychiatry 141:628–632, 1984

Dallman M, Yates FE: Dynamic asymmetries in the corticosteroid feedback path and distribution-metabolism-binding elements of adrenocortical system. Ann NY Acad Sci 156:696–721, 1969

Dallman MF, Akana SF, Cascio CS, et al: Regulation of ACTH secretion: variations on a theme of B. Rec Prog Horm Res 43:113–171, 1987

Dallman MF, Levin N, Cascio CS, et al: Pharmacological evidence that the inhibition of diurnal adrenocorticotropin secretion by corticosteroids is mediated via type I corticosterone-preferring receptors. Endocrinology 124:2844–2850, 1989

Darlington DN, Shinsako J, Dallman MF: Medullary lesions eliminate ACTH responses to hypotensive hemorrhage. Am J Physiol 251:R106–115, 1986

Dave JR, Eiden LE, Lozovsky D, et al: Calcium-independent and calcium-dependent mechanisms regulate corticotropin-releasing factor stimulated proopiomelanocortin peptide secretion and messenger ribonucleic acid production. Endocrinology 120:305–310, 1987

De Souza EB, Insel TR, Perrin MH, et al: Differential regulation of corticotropin-releasing factor receptors in anterior and intermediate lobes of pituitary and brain following adrenalectomy in rats. Neurosci Lett 56:121–128, 1985

DeKloet ER, DeKock S, Schild V, et al: Antiglucocorticoid RU 38486 attenuates retention of a behaviour and disinhibits the hypothalamic-pituitary adrenal axis at different brain sites. Neuroendocrinology 47:109–115, 1988

Dobrakovova M, Kvetnansky R, Torda T, et al: Changes of plasma and adrenal catecholamines and corticosterone in stressed rats with septal lesions. Physiol Behav 29:41–45, 1982

Dolnikoff MS, Kater CE, Egami M, et al: Neonatal treatment with monosodium glutamate increases plasma corticosterone in the rat. Neuroendocrinology 48:645–649, 1988

Dores RM, Jain M, Akil H: Characterization of the forms of β-endorphin and α-MSH in the caudal medulla of the rat and guinea pig. Brain Res 377:251–260, 1986

Dorovini-Zis K, Zis AP: Increase adrenal weight in victims of violent suicide. Am J Psychiatry 144:1214–1215, 1987

Drouin J, Chamberland M, Charron J, et al: Structure of the rat pro-opiomelanocortin (POMC) gene. FEBS Lett 193:54–58, 1985

Dunn JD: Plasma corticosterone responses to electrical stimulation of the bed nucleus of the stria terminalis. Brain Res 407:327–331, 1987

Dunn JD, Orr SE: Differential plasma corticosterone responses to hippocampal stimulation. Exp Brain Res 54:1–6, 1984

Dunn JD, Whitener J: Plasma corticosterone responses to electrical stimulation of the amygdaloid complex: cytoarchitectonic specificity. Neuroendocrinology 42:211–217, 1986

Eberwine JH, Jonassen JA, Evinger MJQ, et al: Complex transcriptional regulation by glucocorticoids and corticotropin releasing hormone of proopiomelanocortin gene expression in rat pituitary cultures. DNA 6:483–492, 1987

Fang VS, Tricou BJ, Robertson A, et al: Plasma ACTH and cortisol levels in depressed patients: relationship to dexamethasone suppression test. Life Sci 29:931–938, 1981

Feldman S: Neural pathways mediating adrenocortical responses. Fed Proc 44:169–175, 1985

Feldman S, Conforti N: Participation of the dorsal hippocampus in the glucocorticoid feedback effect on adrenocortical activity. Neuroendocrinology 30:52–55, 1980

Feldman S, Conforti N: Modifications of adrenocortical responses following frontal cortex stimulation in rats with hypothalamic deafferentations and medial forebrain bundle lesions. Neuroscience 15:1045–1047, 1985

Feldman S, Conforti N, Melamed E: Paraventricular nucleus serotonin mediates neurally stimulated adrenocortical secretion. Brain Res Bull 18:165–168, 1987

Fendler K, Karmos G, Telegdy G: The effect of hippocampal lesion on pituitary-adrenal function. Acta Physiol (Budapest) 20:283–297, 1961

Fischette CT, Komisaruk BR, Edinger HM, et al: Differential fornix ablations and the circadian rhythmicity of adrenal corticosteroid secretion. Brain Res 195:373–387, 1980

Fremeau RT, Lundblat JR, Pritchett DP, et al: Regulation of POMC gene transcription in individual cell nuclei. Science 234:1265–1269, 1986

Fuxe K, Wikström A-C, Okret S, et al: Mapping of glucocorticoid receptor immunoreactive neurons in the rat tel- and diencephalon using a monoclonal antibody against rat liver glucocorticoid receptor. Endocrinology 117:1803–1812, 1985

Gibson A, Hart SL, Patel S: Effects of 6-hydroxydopamine-induced lesions of the paraventricular nucleus, and of prazosin, on the corticosterone response to restraint in rats. Neuropharmacology 25:257–260, 1986

Gold PW, Loriaux DL, Roy A, et al: Response to corticotropin-releasing hormone in the hypercortisolism of depression and Cushing's disease. N Engl J Med 314:1329–1335, 1986

Gray TS, Carney ME, Magnuson DJ: Direct projections from the central amygdaloid nucleus to the hypothalamic paraventricular nucleus: possible role in stress-induced adrenocorticotropin release. Neuroendocrinology 50:433–446, 1989

Halbreich U, Asnis GM, Schindledecker R, et al: Cortisol secretion in endogenous depression, I: basal plasma levels. Arch Gen Psychiatry 42:909–914, 1985

Harbuz MS, Lightman SL: Glucocorticoid inhibition of stress-induced changes in hypothalamic corticotropin releasing factor messenger RNA and proenkephalin A messenger RNA. Neuropeptides 14:17–20, 1989

Hauger RL, Millan MA, Lorang M, et al: Corticotropin releasing factor receptors and pituitary adrenal responses during immobilization stress. Endocrinology 123:396–405, 1988

Herman JP, Schäfer MK-H, Young EA, et al: Evidence for hippocampal regulation of the hypothalamo-pituitary-adrenocortical axis. J Neurosci 9:3072–3082, 1989a

Herman JP, Young EA, Savina A, et al: Hippocampal-hypothalamic circuits mediating tonic inhibition of the hypothalamo-pituitary-adrenocortical (HPA) axis (abstract). Soc Neurosci Abstr 15:135, 1989b

Herman JP, Schäfer MK-H, Sladek CD, et al: Chronic electroconvulsive shock treatment elicits up-regulation of CRH and AVP mRNA in select populations of neuroendocrine neurons. Brain Res 501:235–246, 1989c

Herman JP, Wiegand SW, Watson SW: Regulation of basal corticotropin-releasing hormone and arginine vasopressin in mRNA in the paraventricular nucleus: effects of selective hypothalamic deafferentations. Endocrinology 127:2408–2417, 1990

Hillhouse EW, Jones MT: Effect of bilateral adrenalectomy and corticosteroid therapy on the secretion of corticotropin-releasing factor activity from the hypothalamus of the rat. J Endocrinol 71:21–30, 1976

Hollt V, Przewlocki R, Haarmann I, et al: Stress-induced alterations in the levels of messenger RNA coding for proopiomelanocortin and prolactin in rat pituitary. Neuroendocrinology 43:227–282, 1986

Holsboer F, Doerr HG, Gerken A, et al: Cortisol, 11-deoxycortisol, and ACTH concentration after dexamethasone in depressed patients and healthy volunteers. Psychiatry Res 11:15–23, 1983

Holsboer F, Bardeleden U, Gerken A, et al: Blunted corticotropin and normal cortisol response to human corticotropin-releasing factor in depression. N Engl J Med 311:1127, 1984

Imaki T, Nahon JL, Rivier C, et al: Effect of chronic stress on the level of corticotropin-releasing factor (CRF) mRNA in the rat brain. Soc Neurosci Abstr 14:446, 1988

Ixart G, Barbanel G, Conte-Devolx B, et al: Evidence for basal and stress-induced release of corticotropin releasing factor in the push-pull cannulated median eminence of conscious free moving rats. Neurosci Lett 74:85–89, 1987

Jaeckle RS, López JF: Corticotropin releasing hormone: Clinical endocrinology and implications for Cushing's disease and endogenous depression. Psychiatr Med 3:111–134, 1986

Jaeckle RS, Kathol RG, López JF, et al: Enhanced adrenal sensitivity to exogenous ACTH₁₋₂₄ stimulation in major depression: relationship to dexamethasone suppression test result. Arch Gen Psychiatry 43:233–240, 1987

Jones MT, Brush FR, Neame RLB: Characteristics of fast feedback control of corticotrophin release by corticosteroids. J Endocrinol 55:489–497, 1972

Jones MT, Tiptaft EM, Brush FR: Evidence for dual corticosterone receptor mechanism in the control of adrenocorticotropin secretion. J Endocrinol 60:223–233, 1974

Kalin NH, Weiler SJ, Shelton SE: Plasma ACTH and cortisol concentrations before and after dexamethasone. Psychiatry Res 7:87–92, 1982

Kathol RG, Jaeckle RS, López JF, et al: Pathophysiology of HPA axis abnormalities in patients with major depression: an update. Am J Psychiatry 146:311–317, 1989

Keller-Wood ME, Dallman MF: Corticosteroid inhibition of ACTH secretion. Endocr Rev 5:1–24, 1985

King BM, Dallman MF, Esquerre KR, et al: Radio-frequency vs. electrolytic VMH lesions: differential effects on plasma hormones. Am J Physiol 254:R917–924, 1988

Kiss JZ: Dynamism of chemoarchitecture in the hypothalamic paraventricular nucleus. Brain Res Bull 20:699–708, 1988

Kiss JZ, Mezey E, Skirboll L: Corticotropin releasing-factor neurons of the paraventricular nucleus become vasopressin-positive after adrenalectomy. Proc Natl Acad Sci USA 81:1854–1858, 1984a

Kiss JZ, Cassell MD, Palkovits M: Analysis of the ACTH/B-END/A-MSH-immunoreactive afferent input to the hypothalamic paraventricular nucleus of the rat. Brain Res 324:94–99, 1984b

Knigge KM: Adrenocortical response to stress in rats with lesions in hippocampus and amygdala. Proc Soc Exp Biol Med 108:67–69, 1961

Koch B, Lutz-Bucher B: Specific receptors for vasopressin in the pituitary gland: evidence for down-regulation and desensitization to adrenocorticotropin-releasing factors. Endocrinology 116:671–676, 1985

Kovacs K, Makara GB: Corticosterone and dexamethasone act at different brain sites to inhibit adrenalectomy-induced adrenocorticotropin hypersecretion. Brain Res 474:205–210, 1988

Kovacs K, Mezey E: Dexamethasone inhibits corticotropin releasing factor gene expression in the paraventricular nucleus of the rat. Neuroendocrinology 46:365–368, 1987

Kovacs K, Kiss JZ, Makara GB: Glucocorticoid implants around the hypothalamic paraventricular nucleus prevent the increase of corticotropin-releasing factor and arginine vasopressin immunostaining induced by adrenalectomy. Neuroendocrinology 44:229–234, 1986

Lamberts SWJ, Verleun T, Oosterom R, et al: Corticotropin-releasing factor (ovine) and vasopressin exert a synergistic effect on adrenocorticotropin release in man. J Clin Endocrinol Metab 58:298–303, 1984

Leroux P, Pelletier G: Radiographic study of binding and internalization of corticotropin-releasing factor by rat anterior pituitary corticotrophs. Endocrinology 114:14–21, 1984

Lightman SL, Young WS III: Corticotropin-releasing factor, vasopressin and proopiomelanocortin mRNA responses to stress and opiates in the rat. J Physiol (Lond) 403:511–523, 1987

Lind RW, Swanson LW, Bruhn TO, et al: The distribution of angiotensin II-immunoreactive cells and fibers in the paraventriculo-hypophysial system of the rat. Brain Res 338:81–89, 1985

Linkowski P, Mendlewicz J, Leclercq R, et al: The 24-hour profile of adrenocorticotropin and cortisol in major depressive illness. J Clin Endocrinol Metab 61:429–436, 1985

Linkowski P, Mendlewicz J, Kerkhofs M, et al: 24 hour profiles of ACTH, cortisol and growth hormone in major depressive illness: effect of antidepressant treatment. J Clin Endocrinol Metab 65:141–152, 1987

Loeffler JP, Kley N, Pittius CW, et al: Corticotropin-releasing factor and forskolin increase proopiomelanocortin messenger RNA levels in rat anterior and intermediate cells in vitro. Neurosci Lett 62:383–387, 1985

López JF, Mansour A, Akil H, et al: Localization of POMC mRNA, glucocorticoid receptor mRNA and CRF receptors in human pituitaries. Soc Neurosci Abstr 14:1275, 1988

Lundblad JR, Roberts JL: Regulation of proopiomelanocortin gene expression in pituitary. Endocr Rev 9:135–158, 1988

Magariños AM, Somoza G, DeNicola AF: Glucocorticoid negative feedback and glucocorticoid receptors after hippocampectomy in rats. Horm Metab Res 19:105–109, 1987

Makara GB, Stark E, Karteszi M, et al: Effects of paraventricular lesions on stimulated ACTH release and CRF in stalk-median eminence of rat. Am J Physiol 240:E441–446, 1981

Matthews J, Akil H, Greden J, et al: β-endorphin/β-lipotropin immunoreactivity in endogenous depression. Arch Gen Psychiatry 43:374–381, 1986

McKnight SL, Kingsbury R: Transcriptional control signals of a eucaryotic protein-coding gene. Science 217:316–324, 1982

Merchenthaler I, Hynes MA, Vigh S, et al: Corticotropin-releasing factor (CRF): origin and course of afferent pathways to the median eminence (ME) of the rat hypothalamus. Neuroendocrinology 39:296–306, 1983

Mezey E, Kiss JZ, Skirboll LR, et al: Increase of corticotropin-releasing factor staining in rat paraventricular nucleus neurons by depletion of hypothalamic adrenaline. Nature 310:140–141, 1984

Miyazki K, Reisine T, Kebabian JW: Adenosine 3', 5'-monophosphate (cAMP) dependent protein kinase activity in rodent pituitary tissue: possible role in cAMP dependent hormone secretion. Endocrinology 115:1933–1945, 1984

Moberg GP, Scapagnini V, DeGroot J, et al: Effect of sectioning the fornix on diurnal fluctuations in plasma corticosterone levels in the rat. Neuroendocrinology 7:11–15, 1971

Moore RY, Eichler VB: Loss of a circadian adrenocortical rhythm following suprachiasmatic lesions in the rat. Brain Res 42:201–206, 1972

Nakamura N, Nakanishi S, Sueoka S, et al: Effects of steroid hormones on the level of corticotropin messenger RNA activity in cultured mouse-pituitary-tumor cell. Eur J Biochem 86:61–66, 1978

Nasr SJ, Rodgers C, Pandey G, et al: ACTH and the dexamethasone suppression test in depression. Biol Psychiatry 18:1069–1073, 1983

Negro-Vilar A, Johnston C, Spinedi E, et al: Physiological role of peptides and amines on the regulation of ACTH secretion. Ann NY Acad Sci 512:218–236, 1987

Nelson DH: Cushing's syndrome, in Endocrinology, Vol 2. Edited by DeGroot LJ. Philadelphia, PA, WB Saunders, 1989, pp 1660–1675

Nemeroff CB, Owens MJ, Bissette G, et al: Reduced corticotropin releasing factor binding sites in the frontal cortex of suicide victims. Arch Gen Psychiatry 45:577–579, 1984

Norman TR, Piperoglou M, McIntyre IM, et al: Plasma immunoreactive β-endorphin in dexamethasone suppressors and non-suppressors of cortisol. J Affective Disord 12:233–239, 1987

Nyakas C, DeKloet ER, Bohus B: Hippocampal function and putative corticosterone receptors: effect of septal lesions. Neuroendocrinology 29:301–312, 1979

Oldfield BJ, Silverman A-J: A light microscopic HRP study of limbic projections to the vasopressin-containing nuclear groups of the hypothalamus. Brain Res Bull 14:143–157, 1985

Perrin MH, Haas Y, Rivier JE, et al: Corticotropin-releasing factor binding to the anterior pituitary receptor is modulated by divalent cations and guanyl nucleotides. Endocrinology 118:1171–1179, 1986

Pfohl B, Sherman B, Schlecte J, et al: Pituitary-adrenal axis rhythm disturbance in psychiatric depression. Arch Gen Psychiatry 42:897–903, 1985a

Pfohl B, Sherman B, Schlechte J, et al: Differences in plasma ACTH and cortisol between depressed patients and normal controls. Biol Psychiatry 20:1055–1072, 1985b

Piekut DT, Joseph SA: Relationship of CRF-immunostained cells and magnocellular neurons in the paraventricular nucleus of rat hypothalamus. Peptides 6:873–882, 1985

Plotsky PM: Facilitation of immunoreactive corticotropin-releasing factor secretion into the hypophysial-portal circulation after activation of catecholaminergic pathways or central norepinephrine injection. Endocrinology 121:924–930, 1987a

Plotsky PM: Regulation of hypophysiotropic factors mediating ACTH secretion. Ann NY Acad Sci 512:205–217, 1987b

Raymond V, Leung PCK, Veilleux R, et al: Vasopressin rapidly stimulates phosphatidic acid-phosphatidylinositol turnover in rat anterior pituitary cells. FEBS Lett 182:196–200, 1985

Reisine T, Rougon G, Barbet J, et al: Corticotropin-releasing factor induced adrenocorticotropin hormone release and synthesis is blocked by incorporation of the inhibitor of cyclic AMP-dependent protein kinase into anterior pituitary cells by liposomes. Proc Natl Acad Sci USA 82:8261–8265, 1985

Reul JMHM, DeKloet ER: Differential response of type I and type II corticosteroid receptors to changes in plasma steroid level and circadian rhythmicity. Neuroendocrinology 45:407–412, 1987

Reus VI, Joseph MS, Dallman MF: ACTH levels after the dexamethasone suppression test in depression. N Engl J Med 306:238–239, 1982

Risch SC: Beta-endorphin hypersecretion: possible cholinergic mechanism. Biol Psychiatry 17:1071–1079, 1982

Rivier C, Vale W: Influence of the frequency of corticotropin releasing factor administration on adrenocorticotropin and corticosterone secretion in rat. Endocrinology 113:1422–1427, 1983

Roberts JL, Budarf MJ, Baxter JD, et al: Selective reduction of proadrenocorticotropin/endorphin protein and messenger ribonucleic acid activity in mouse pituitary tumor cells by glucocorticoids. Biochem 18:4907–4915, 1979a

Roberts JL, Johnson LK, Baxter JD, et al: Effect of glucocorticoids on the synthesis and processing of the common precursor to adrenocorticotropin and endorphin in mouse pituitary tumor cells, in Hormones and Cell Culture, Book B. Edited by Sato GH, Ross R. Cold Spring Harbor, NY, Cold Spring Harbor Laboratory Press, 1979b, pp 827–842

Rubin RT, Poland RE, Lesser IM, et al: Neuroendocrine aspects of primary endogenous depression, I: cortisol secretory dynamics in patients and matched controls. Arch Gen Psychiatry 44:328–336, 1987

Rupprecht R, Barocka A, Beck G, et al: Pre- and postdexamethasone plasma ACTH and β-endorphin levels in endogenous and nonendogenous depression. Biol Psychiatry 23:531–535, 1988

Sachar EJ, Hellman L, Roffwarg HP, et al: Disrupted 24 hour patterns of cortisol secretion in psychotic depressives. Arch Gen Psychiatry 28:19–24, 1973

Sakly M, Koch B: Ontogenesis of glucocorticoid receptors in anterior pituitary gland: transient dissociation among cytoplasmic receptor density, nuclear uptake and regulation of corticotropic activity. Endocrinology 108:591–596, 1981

Saphier D, Feldman S: Effects of neural stimuli on paraventricular nucleus neurons. Brain Res Bull 14:401–407, 1985

Saphier D, Feldman S: Effects of septal and hippocampal stimuli on paraventricular nucleus neurons. Neuroscience 20:749–755, 1987

Saphier D, Feldman S: Iontophoretic application of glucocorticoids inhibits identified neurons in the rat paraventricular nucleus. Brain Res 453:183–190, 1988

Sapolsky RM, Krey LC, McEwen BS: Glucocorticoid-sensitive hippocampal neurons are involved in terminating the adrenocortical stress response. Proc Natl Acad Sci USA 81:6174–6177, 1984

Sapolsky RM, Krey LC, McEwen BS: The neuroendocrinology of stress and aging: the glucocorticoid cascade hypothesis. Endocr Rev 7:284–301, 1986

Sawchenko PE: Adrenalectomy-induced enhancement of CRF and vasopressin immunoreactivity in parvocellular neurosecretory neurons: anatomic, peptide and steroid specificity. J Neurosci 7:1093–1106, 1987a

Sawchenko PE: Evidence for a local site of action for glucocorticoids in inhibiting CRF and vasopressin expression in the paraventricular nucleus. Brain Res 403:213–224, 1987b

Sawchenko PE: Effects of catecholamine-depleting medullary knife cuts on corticotropin-releasing factor and vasopressin immunoreactivity in the hypothalamus of normal and ateroid-manipulated rats. Neuroendocrinology 48:459–470, 1988

Sawchenko PE, Swanson LW: The organization of forebrain afferents to the paraventricular and supraoptic nuclei of the rat. J Comp Neurol 218:121–144, 1983

Sawchenko PE, Swanson LW, Steinbusch HWM, et al: The distribution and cells of origin of serotonin inputs to the paraventricular and supraoptic nuclei of the rat. Brain Res 277:355–360, 1983

Sawchenko PE, Swanson LW, Vale WW: Co-expression of corticotropin-releasing factor and vasopressin immunoreactivity in parvocellular neurosecretory neurons of the adrenalectomized rat. Proc Natl Acad Sci USA 81:1883–1887, 1984

Sawchenko PE, Swanson LW, Grzanna R, et al: Colocalization of neuropeptide Y immunoreactivity in brainstem catecholaminergic neurons that project to the paraventricular and supraoptic nuclei in the rat. J Comp Neurol 241:138–153, 1985

Schachter BS, Johnson LK, Baxter JD, et al: Differential regulation by glucocorticoids of proopiomelanocortin mRNA levels in the anterior and intermediate lobes of the rat pituitary. Endocrinology 110:1442–1444, 1982

Schäfer MK-H, Herman JP, Young EA, et al: Gene expression of neuropeptides related to CRF after adrenalectomy. Soc Neurosci Abstr 13:583, 1987

Scheidereit C, Westphal HM, Carlson C, et al: Molecular model of the interaction between glucocorticoid receptor and the regulatory elements of inducible genes. DNA 5:383–391, 1986

Schwartz J, Billestrup N, Perrin M, et al: Identification of corticotropin releasing factor target cells and effects of dexamethasone on binding in anterior pituitary using a fluorescent analog of CRF. Endocrinology 119:2376–2382, 1986

Seggie J, Uhlir I, Brown GM: Adrenal stress responses following septal lesions in the rat. Neuroendocrinology 16:225–236, 1974

Shiomi H, Watson SJ, Kelsey JE, et al: Pretranslational and posttranslational mechanisms for regulating β-endorphin/ACTH cells: studies in anterior lobe. Endocrinology 119:1793–1799, 1986

Siegel R, Chowers I, Confroni N, et al: Corticotrophin and corticosterone secretory patterns following acute neurogenic stress, in intact rats and variously hypothalamic deafferented rats. Brain Res 188:399–410, 1980

Silverman A-J, Hou-Yu A, Chen W-P: Corticotropin-releasing factor synapses within the paraventricular nucleus of the hypothalamus. Neuroendocrinology 49:291–299, 1989

Swanson LW, Sawchenko PE: Hypothalamic integration: organization of the paraventricular and supraoptic nuclei. Ann Rev Neurosci 6:275–325, 1983

Swanson LW, Köhler C, Björklund A: The limbic region, I: the septohippocampal system, in Handbook of Chemical Neuroanatomy, Vol 5: Integrated Systems of the CNS, Part I. Edited by Björklund A, Hökfelt T, Swanson LW. Amsterdam, Elsevier, 1987, pp 125–278

Szafarczyk A, Ixart G, Malaval F, et al: Effects of lesions of the suprachiasmatic nuclei and *p*-chlorophenylalanine on the circadian rhythms of adrenocorticotropic hormone and corticosterone in the plasma and on locomotor activity of rats. J Endocrinol 83:1–16, 1979

Szafarczyk A, Alonso G, Izart I, et al: Serotonin system and circadian rhythms of ACTH and corticosterone in rats. Am J Physiol 239:482–489, 1980a

Szafarczyk A, Hery M, Laplante E, et al: Temporal relationships between the circadian rhythmicity in plasma levels of pituitary hormones and in hypothalamic concentrations of releasing factors. Neuroendocrinology 30:369–376, 1980b

Szafarczyk A, Malaval F, Laurent A, et al: Further evidence for a central stimulatory action of catecholamines on adrenocorticotropin release in the rat. Endocrinology 121:883–892, 1987

Szafarczyk A, Guillaume V, Conte-Devolx B, et al: Central catecholaminergic system stimulates secretion of CRH at different sites. Am J Physiol 255:E463–468, 1988

Ter Horst GJ, Luiten PGM: Phaseolus vulgaris leuco-agglutinin tracing of intrahypothalamic connections of the lateral, ventromedial, dorsomedial and paraventricular hypothalamic nuclei in the rat. Brain Res Bull 18:91–203, 1987

Usher DR, Lieblich I, Siegel RA: Pituitary-adrenal function after small and large lesions in the lateral septal area in food-deprived rats. Neuroendocrinology 16:156–164, 1974

Vale W, Spiess J, Rivier C, et al: Characterization of a 41-residue ovine hypothalamic peptide that stimulates secretion of corticotropin and β-endorphin. Science 21:1394–1397, 1981

Watson SJ, Sherman TG, Kelsey JE, et al: Anatomical localization of mRNA: In situ hybridization of neuropeptide systems, in In Situ Hybridization: Applications to Neurobiology. Edited by Valentino K, Eberwine J, Barchas J. New York, Oxford University Press, 1987, pp 126–146

Watts AG, Swanson LW: Diurnal variations in the content of preprocorticotropin-releasing hormone messenger ribonucleic acid in the hypothalamic paraventricular nucleus of both sexes as measured by in situ hybridization. Endocrinology 125:1734–1738, 1989

Whitnall MH: Distribution of pro-vasopressin expressing and pro-vasopressin deficient CRH neurons in the paraventricular hypothalamic nucleus of colchicine-treated normal and adrenalectomized rats. J Comp Neurol 275:13–28, 1988

Whitnall MH, Smyth D, Gainer H: Vasopressin coexists in half of the corticotropin-releasing factor axons present in the external zone of the median eminence in normal rats. Neuroendocrinology 45:420–424, 1987a

Whitnall MH, Key S, Gainer H: Vasopressin-containing and vasopressin-deficient subpopulations of corticotropin-releasing factor axons are differentially affected by adrenalectomy. Endocrinology 120:2180–2182, 1987b

Widmaier EP, Dallman MF: Rapid inhibition and stimulation of ACTH by glucocorticoids in vitro. Fed Proc 42:458, 1983

Wilson MM, Greer SE, Greer MA, et al: Hippocampal inhibition of pituitary-adrenocortical function in female rats. Brain Res 197:433–441, 1980

Winokur G, Pfohl B, Sherman B: The relationship of historically defined subtypes of depression to ACTH and cortisol levels in depression: preliminary study. Biol Psychiatry 20:751–757, 1985

Yerevanian BI, Woolf PD: Plasma ACTH levels in primary depression: relationship to the dexamethasone suppression test. Psychiatry Res 9:319–327, 1983

Yerevanian BI, Woolf PD, Iker HP: Plasma ACTH levels in depression before and after recovery: relationship to the dexamethasone suppression test. Psychiatry Res 10:175–181, 1983

Young EA, Akil H: CRF stimulation of ACTH/beta-endorphin release: effect of acute and chronic stress. Endocrinology 117:23–30, 1985

Young EA, Akil H: Paradoxical effect of corticosteroids on pituitary ACTH/β-endorphin release in stressed animals. Psychoneuroendocrinology 13:317–323, 1988

Young EA, Akana S, Dallman MF: Decreased sensitivity to glucocorticoid fast feedback in chronically stressed rats. Neuroendocrinology 51:536–542, 1990a

Young E, Watson SJ, Kotun J, et al: Response to low dose oCRH in endogenous depression: role of cortisol feedback. Arch Gen Psychiatry 47:449–457, 1990b

Young WS III, Mezey E, Siegel RE: Quantitative in situ hybridization histochemistry reveals increased levels of corticotropin-releasing factor mRNA after adrenalectomy in rats. Neurosci Lett 70:198–203, 1986

Chapter 2

Animal Studies Implicating a Role of Corticotropin-Releasing Hormone in Mediating Behavior Associated With Psychopathology

Ned H. Kalin, M.D., Lorey K. Takahashi, Ph.D.

R esearch has demonstrated that corticotropin-releasing hormone (CRH), a 41–amino acid peptide located in the paraventricular nucleus of the hypothalamus, plays a major role in the regulation of pituitary adrenocorticotropin (ACTH) release (Spiess et al. 1981; Vale et al. 1981). Located primarily in the parvocellular region of the paraventricular nucleus, these CRH neurons project to the median eminence of the hypothalamus where they influence the activity of adenohypophysial cells via the hypothalamic-hypophysial portal system (Antoni et al. 1983; Cummings et al. 1983; Liposits et al. 1983; Merchenthaler et al. 1983).

In addition to its endocrine function, CRH and its receptors are found in extrahypothalamic areas, including the cortex, brainstem, and limbic system (Bloom et al. 1982; Bugnon et al. 1982; De Souza et al. 1984, 1985; Fischman and Muldow 1982; Olschowka et al. 1982a, 1982b). These and other data suggest that CRH may act as a neurotransmitter outside of the hypothalamus (Smith et al. 1986). Experiments suggest that this nonpituitary, extrahypothalamic role of CRH is important in mediating autonomic activation (Brown and Fisher 1983; Brown et al. 1982, 1985; Fisher et al. 1982; Swanson et al. 1983) and electrical brain activity (Aldenhoff et al. 1983; Ehlers et al. 1983). In addition, intracerebroventricular (ICV) administration of CRH, or its receptor antagonist, significantly alters the overt

This work was supported by PHS Grants MH-40855 and DK-35641 and by the Veterans Administration. We thank Steven Shelton, Jack Sherman, Kathleen Renk, Helen Van Valkenburg, Jennifer Vander Burgt, and Eric Baker for technical assistance. We also gratefully acknowledge the skilled assistance of Dee Jones in preparing the manuscript.

display of stress-induced behavior (Berridge and Dunn 1986; Britton et al. 1982; Kalin et al. 1983a; Koob and Bloom 1985; Sutton et al. 1982; Takahashi and Kalin 1989).

From a clinical perspective, interest in CRH stems from the fact that activation of the hypothalamic-pituitary-adrenal (HPA) system occurs in response to stress, and alterations of this system are frequent in depressed patients. The action of CRH in the brain in altering not only endocrine function but also electrophysiological and behavioral activity suggests a potentially significant role of this neuropeptide in mediating the nonendocrine aspects of depression as well as other psychiatric illnesses. In this chapter, we review studies performed in our laboratories investigating the role of CRH in mediating stress-induced behavior in the laboratory rat and the rhesus monkey. This comparative approach may clarify and strengthen the involvement of CRH in mediating the normal and pathological expression of behavior.

RODENT STUDIES

Role of CRH in Mediating Shock-Induced Freezing

Animals, including humans, often exhibit behavioral inhibition when confronted with threatening stimuli whose whereabouts or characteristics are ambiguous or uncertain. An extreme form of behavioral inhibition is commonly referred to as *freezing*, which can be described as the immediate cessation of all body movements except that required for respiration. Animal studies indicate that freezing reduces the risk of attracting the attention of a predator or an aggressive individual until there is an opportunity to escape from the threatening situation or until the danger passes.

In rats, freezing is readily elicited after administration of brief foot shock. Furthermore, freezing is a function of shock intensity—the more intense the shock, the longer the duration of freezing. Thus, by quantifying the duration of freezing, it becomes possible to infer the degree of danger or threat that the animal perceives in the test situation.

As indicated before, ICV administration of CRH was suggested to potentiate the occurrence of stress-induced behavioral and physiological responses. Thus, we hypothesized that ICV administration of CRH would increase the occurrence of shock-induced freezing (Sherman and Kalin 1988). Rats received an ICV injection of 100 or 300 ng of CRH. Control rats were treated with an ICV injection of vehicle. All animals were then placed in an environment where they were shocked or left undisturbed. Before the onset of foot shock, rats seldom froze, and in CRH-treated animals that were left undisturbed, CRH did not significantly increase the occurrence of freezing during the entire test period (Figure 2-1). In contrast, the application of shock rapidly facilitated freezing in all animals. More important, those rats that received the 300-ng dose of CRH exhibited the highest level of freezing. Although the 100-ng dose of CRH also tended to potentiate the display of shock-induced freezing, the level of freezing was not significantly higher than that shown by vehicle-treated rats. Thus, CRH appears to augment the expression of shock-induced freezing in a dose-dependent manner.

Although these results suggest a role of CRH in altering the degree of threat or stress that is perceived by the animal, it is important to determine whether this increase in freezing was mediated directly via CRH systems or indirectly by decreasing pain thresholds to the shock. Therefore, tests to evaluate alterations in pain sensitivity were administered to rats that received ICV injections of either 300 ng CRH or vehicle. These pain-sensitivity tests, administered immediately after exposure to foot shock, indicated that the increased occurrence of shock-induced freezing produced by CRH was not mediated by a heightened response to painful stimuli. These results strengthened the hypothesis that the action of CRH mediates the perception or psychological aspects governing the organism's response to stressors. These results, however, based on exogenously administered CRH, do not necessarily implicate a role of endogenous physiological CRH action in mediating stress-induced behavioral responses.

To directly implicate the action of endogenous CRH in mediating the expression of behavior induced by threat, we next examined the effects of α-helical CRH(9-41), a specific synthetic competitive antagonist of the CRH receptor, on shock-induced freezing (Kalin et al. 1989). In this study, we predicted that antagonism of CRH receptors would reduce the occurrence of shock-induced freezing.

Rats received ICV injections of α-helical CRH(9-41) at doses of 0, 5, or 25 μg. The 25-μg dose was found to be the most effective in reducing the expression of shock-induced freezing. It is important that the CRH antagonist produced no significant alteration in the animal's sensitivity to pain (Figure 2-2).

The implications of these results are twofold. First, they strongly implicate an involvement of endogenous CRH in mediating the acute display of stress-induced behavior. Second, CRH produced alterations in the expression of stress-induced behavior are mediated through mechanisms other than those that influence the perception of pain.

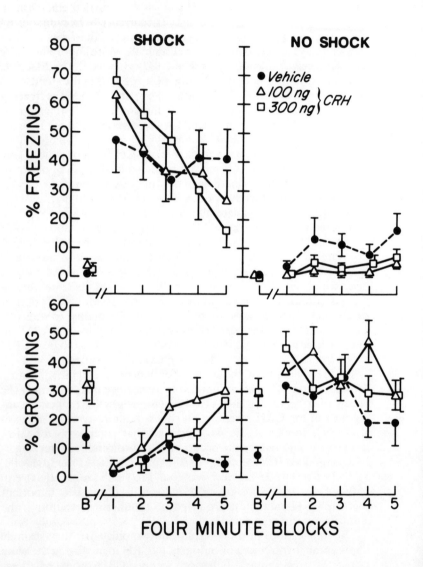

Figure 2-1. Mean percent ± SE of freezing and grooming scored for each 4-minute block of testing at baseline (B) and postbaseline. CRH, corticotropin-releasing hormone.

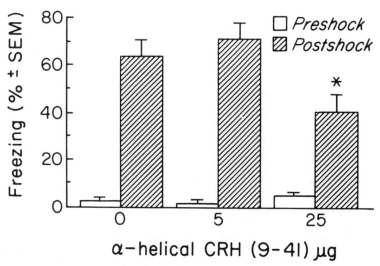

Figure 2-2. Effects of intracerebroventricular infusion of corticotropin-releasing hormone (CRH) receptor antagonist on preshock and postshock freezing (mean ± SE). *$P < .05$; significantly different from 0- and 5-μg postshock groups.

Effects of α-Helical CRH(9-41) on Mediating Freezing Induced by Prior Shock Experiences

In an animal the association between an environment and its level of danger forms rapidly and lasts long. Memory of specific threats occurring in particular locations must have been selected at a premium, because the cost of forgetting can be lethal. Hence, prey species tend to regulate their behavioral activities by avoiding habitats associated with predators or, if necessary, traverse the dangerous habitat as inconspicuously and as rapidly as possible. In the latter situation, the animal is highly aroused even when danger is not readily apparent. As shown by laboratory studies, animals that are returned to an environment associated with shock exhibit a significant activation in autonomic and endocrinological systems. In addition, the behavior of rats that are reexposed to the environment previously associated with shock can be characterized as fearful or defensive, as evidenced by a heightened level of freezing.

We examined whether the action of endogenous CRH was also involved in the display of freezing induced by psychological stress (Kalin and Takahashi 1990). The testing procedure involved the administration of foot shock in an unfamiliar environment on day 1. Immediately after shock, the rats were returned to their living quarters. On day 2, they received an ICV infusion of either 20 μg of α-helical CRH(9-41) or vehicle before reexposure to the shock environment. With these test conditions, antagonist-treated rats exhibited a significant reduction in freezing duration (Table 2-1).

We also examined whether α-helical CRH(9-41) was involved in attenuating freezing through its action in hypothalamic regions that mediate pituitary ACTH secretion (Table 2-1). The elevation in plasma ACTH concentrations, measured immediately after reexposure to the environment associated with shock, was not significantly different between antagonist-treated and control rats. This result suggests that CRH action that mediates freezing probably occurs in extrahypothalamic brain regions.

In summary, these studies strongly suggest a role of endogenous CRH in mediating the expression of defensive behavior elicited by painful stimuli or a psychologically stressful environment. It is important that the behavioral effects produced by endogenous CRH action do not appear to be mediated by peripheral pituitary-adrenal hormones or by an indirect alteration in nociceptive processes.

Role of CRH Systems in Mediating Behavior Induced by Psychological Stress in a Seminaturalistic Environment

We believed it would be important to examine the generality of the role of CRH in mediating the expression of defensive behavior induced by psychological stress. Consequently, we developed a testing paradigm that would not rely on the administration of electric shock to induce anxiety but would mimic anxiety-producing situations that a free-ranging animal would encounter in its natural environment (Takahashi et al. 1989).

Table 2-1. Effects of intracerebroventricular infusion of 20 μg of α-helical CRH (9-41) or vehicle on behavioral responses (s) and plasma ACTH induced by 15-minute reexposure to shock box

Measure	Vehicle	α-helical CRH(9-41)
Freeze	458 ± 72	266 ± 52*
Crouch	127 ± 17	176 ± 20
Walk/rear	186 ± 44	306 ± 57
Groom	43 ± 16	37 ± 7
ACTH (pg/ml)	185 ± 81	134 ± 33

Note. Values are means ± SE.
*$P < .05$; significantly different from vehicle group.

The test apparatus involved a small darkened chamber that opened into a large, brightly lit arena. Rats placed initially into the unfamiliar small chamber seldom ventured into the large arena, preferring to spend most of their time remaining inconspicuous within the darkened chamber. This initial reticence to emerge from the protective confines of the chamber probably reflects the rats' assessment of the degree of threat, such as predators that may be lurking in an unfamiliar environment. However, as an animal becomes familiar with its environment, by reexposing it to the apparatus on the next day, it emerges from the small chamber to explore the large arena. Presumably, the absence of a clear identifiable threat lessens the stressful impact of an unfamiliar situation and promotes behavioral responses that are more interactive with the environment. In nature, exploration of an unfamiliar but nonthreatening habitat may lead to increased acquisition of resources, such as food or shelter.

This transition from an initial withdrawal reaction to a subsequent exploration of the unfamiliar environment was studied in our laboratory by using the CRH receptor antagonist and agonist. To determine whether endogenous CRH action was involved in mediating behavioral responses in the test situation, we first examined whether ICV administration of α-helical CRH(9-41) would reduce a rat's perception of threat in the unfamiliar environment. We reasoned that a reduction in anxiety would be manifested by increased exploration of the large unfamiliar arena when the animal is placed for the first time in the small chamber. As we show in Table 2-2, antagonist-treated rats had significantly shorter latencies to emerge from the small protective chamber, spent less time in the chamber, and made frequent passages between the chamber and the large arena.

On the basis of these observations, which implicated the importance of endogenous CRH action, we then hypothesized that ICV injections of CRH would produce increased anxiety and reverse the tendency to explore the open environment on the rats' second

Table 2-2. Effect of 20 μg of α-helical CRH(9-41) on defensive withdrawal and exploratory behavior

Treatment	Latency to leave chamber (s)	Time in chamber per entry (s)	Number of passages
Vehicle	693 ± 109	671 ± 115	1.8 ± 1.0
α-helical CRH(9-41)	158 ± 64**	139 ± 48**	12.8 ± 2.7*

Note. Values are means ± SE.
*P <.01, **P <.001; significantly different from vehicle group.

exposure to the test apparatus. Therefore, in this study, rats were preexposed to the test situation by placing them in the small chamber located in the large arena. The next day, rats received an ICV injection of either CRH (300 ng) or vehicle and returned to the small chamber. Whereas vehicle-treated rats spent more time exploring the large arena on their second experience, CRH-treated rats spent most of their time withdrawn in the chamber. As we show in Figure 2-3, CRH injections significantly increased the latency to leave the chamber, increased the amount of time spent in the chamber, and decreased the number of passages made between the protective chamber and the open arena. These results suggest that ICV administration of CRH increased the animals' degree of anxiety, thereby reducing exploratory or interactive tendencies with the open environment.

Additional studies were conducted using this model of psychological stress. Results of this research suggest that the action of CRH is mediated in the brain and not through peripheral hormonal effects and that CRH-treated rats, presumably anxiety prone, will initiate responses to enter the protective chamber when placed in the center of the large arena. Taken together, antagonism of endogenous CRH receptors produces a decrease in withdrawal and an increase in environmental exploration. In contrast, exogenous administration of CRH heightens the withdrawal reaction in a partly familiar environment that contains no recognizable threat.

Role of CRH in Mediating Fear-Motivated Behavior Induced by Odors of Stressed Conspecifics

Although our earlier studies implicated endogenous CRH systems in the mediation of defensive behavior induced by foot shock and an unfamiliar open field, a role of endogenous CRH in mediating responses activated by a biologically relevant stressor would significantly advance the generality of our earlier results. The studies reported in this section examine whether the action of endogenous CRH is involved in the mediation of behavior induced by a stressor that a rat may confront during exploration of its natural habitat.

Rodents have evolved with a highly developed olfactory system that is used to obtain information about the environment. One important use of this olfactory system is to acquire information concerning the extent of environmental danger. For example, rats will respond to odors of urine and feces made by other stressed rats by rapidly engaging in protective behavior. Withdrawal from a habitat marked by cues indicative of recent distress may be very important in facilitating survival in a small mammal.

To examine the involvement of endogenous CRH receptors in the

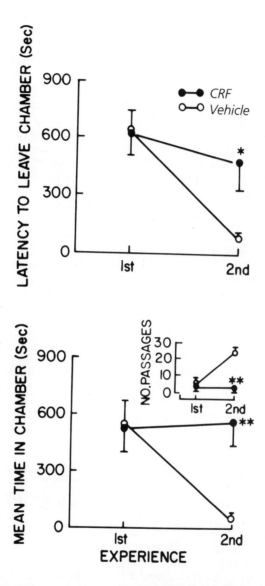

Figure 2-3.   Mean ± SE occurrence of behavioral responses exhibited after intracerebroventricular injection of 300 ng corticotropin-releasing hormone (CRF) or vehicle 20 minutes before second test. Rats were placed in small chamber at start of each test. *$P < .05$, **$P < .01$; significantly different from vehicle group.

expression of behavior induced by odors associated with stress, we preexposed rats to the large arena containing the small darkened chamber (Takahashi et al. 1990). The next day, rats received an ICV infusion of either 20 μg of α-helical CRH(9-41) or vehicle. Immediately before reexposure testing, urine and feces from a stressed conspecific were collected on a cardboard sheet and placed in a corner of the large open arena. Both vehicle- and antagonist-treated rats rapidly withdrew into the small chamber when reexposed to the open arena containing the odors (Figure 2-4). However, unlike vehicle-treated rats, which, for the most part, remained hidden in the chamber during the entire test period, antagonist-treated rats emerged from the chamber to explore the arena.

These results are not only significant in implicating the action of endogenous CRH receptors in mediating behavior induced by a natural stressor; they also raise the intriguing hypothesis that a decrease in CRH action may be as detrimental to an animal as an increase. That is, results of this study suggest that antagonist-treated rats respond inappropriately to a potentially dangerous situation by exposing themselves to an environment marked with social cues indicating the possible presence of a predator or a hostile conspecific.

MONKEY STUDIES

The rhesus monkey is a highly social old-world monkey, and numerous similarities in behavioral and physiological systems exist between the rhesus monkey and humans. Extensive studies have been performed validating models of stress and psychopathology in this species. Therefore, studies that use the rhesus monkey provide a unique opportunity to explore mechanisms underlying human psychopathology (McKinney 1977).

Effects of CRH on the Infant Monkey's Response to Brief Maternal Separation

Infant-maternal separation or attachment bond disruption is a common occurrence in humans. In vulnerable individuals, however, separation from the mother may induce or exacerbate the expression of psychopathology. When infant monkeys are separated from their mothers, they respond by emitting coo vocalizations and increasing their activity levels (Kalin and Carnes 1984). These behaviors have been hypothesized to facilitate retrieval of the infant by its mother. If an infant is separated from its mother and perceives a threat in the environment, however, a common response is to inhibit its activity (Kalin and Shelton 1989). It is believed that, similar to freezing in the rat, the monkey's behavioral inhibition may serve a protective func-

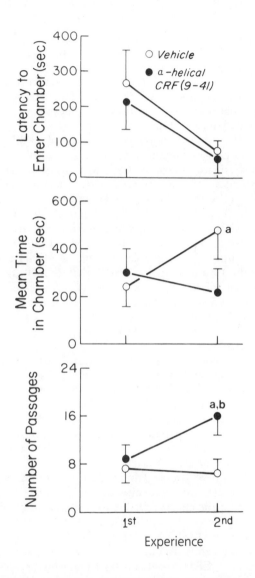

Figure 2-4. Mean ± SE occurrence of behavioral responses exhibited after intracerebroventricular injection of corticotropin-releasing hormone receptor antagonist α-helical CRF(9-41) or vehicle 20 minutes before second test. Rats were placed in center of large arena containing odors of stressed conspecifics at start of each test. [a]$P < .05$, significantly different from first experience. [b]$P < .05$, significantly different from vehicle group.

tion. Separation also results in activation of HPA (Gunnar et al. 1981; Kalin et al. 1988a) and autonomic systems (Reite and Short 1978). These physiological changes provide metabolic support for the infant in the mother's absence. Our primate laboratory has been investigating the neurochemical systems that mediate behavioral and hormonal changes that occur in infant rhesus monkeys during a brief period of maternal separation. Our earlier work established that opiate (Kalin et al. 1988a) and benzodiazepine (Kalin et al. 1987a) systems modulate the response of infant monkeys to separation.

To investigate the role of CRH systems in mediating the infant's response to separation, we separated 11 infant monkeys from their mothers and treated them at weekly intervals with one of four doses of CRH—0, .5, 1.0, or 10.0 µg (Kalin et al. 1989). Each animal was exposed to all four doses, which were administered ICV. At the conclusion of the separation period, blood samples were collected from the infants for the measurement of ACTH and cortisol concentrations. Results demonstrated that the 10-µg dose of CRH reduced an infant's level of locomotion, increased the amount of inactivity, and had no effect on coo vocalizations (Figure 2-5). In addition, this dose of CRH significantly increased ACTH and cortisol levels. It is important that these changes occurred without sedating the animals.

These findings are of interest because our earlier work demonstrated that an anti-anxiety compound increased (Kalin et al. 1987a) and an anxiogenic agent decreased (unpublished observations) the activity levels of separated infants. Specifically, we found that diazepam increased locomotion and reduced ACTH levels in infants undergoing brief separation. In contrast, administration of the benzodiazepine inverse agonist β-CCE had effects similar to CRH by reducing infants' activity levels.

Intracerebroventricular administration of a compound can result in leakage of the substance into the periphery. Therefore, to demonstrate that the effects of CRH were mediated by direct actions on the central nervous system and not through peripheral mechanisms, we administered vehicle or 10 µg CRH intravenously to monkeys (Kalin et al. 1989). In contrast to ICV administration, peripherally administered CRH produced no significant behavioral effects. In addition, after peripheral administration, this dose of CRH was not as potent in stimulating ACTH secretion as the same dose administered ICV.

Effects of Higher Doses of CRH Administered to Adult Monkeys

To assess the effects of higher doses of CRH, we performed studies in adult rhesus monkeys (Kalin et al. 1983b). In the first study, four partially restrained adult male monkeys received ICV injections of vehicle or CRH (20 and 180 µg). As we found with the lower doses, these doses resulted in significant increases in plasma concentrations of ACTH and cortisol. In addition, a slight increase in mean arterial blood pressure was observed. Compared with vehicle, CRH resulted in behavioral arousal. Increases in vocalizations, head shaking, and struggling occurred.

We next administered CRH to the same monkeys while they were moving freely in their home cages. In this environment, CRH induced a very different behavioral response. Vocalizations were increased after both 20 and 180 µg of CRH. The 180-µg dose resulted in behavioral

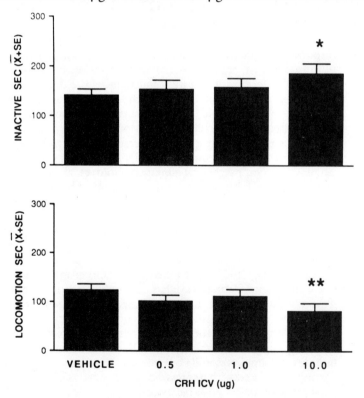

Figure 2-5. Effects of intracerebroventricular (ICV)-administered corti-cotropin-releasing hormone (CRH) on activity levels of 11 infant rhesus monkeys. *$P < .05$, significantly different from vehicle. **$P < .01$, significantly different from vehicle.

inhibition characterized by huddling and lying down behaviors (Figure 2-6).

These effects were not caused by sedation because, when approached by a human, the animals responded normally. The results also cannot be explained by a reduction in blood pressure, because in the earlier experiment we demonstrated that this dose of CRH resulted in a small blood pressure increase. The CRH-induced huddling behavior appeared to be remarkably similar to behaviors induced in infants undergoing long-term separations (Harlow and Suomi 1974). This is of interest because huddling in monkeys has been specifically linked to behavioral despair and depression.

PUTATIVE ROLE OF CRH SYSTEMS IN MEDIATING PSYCHOPATHOLOGY

Activation of the HPA system is an important aspect of the stress response and is frequently accompanied by behavioral changes. Under normal circumstances, stress-induced activation of behavioral and hormonal responses is adaptive and reduces the deleterious consequences of the stressor. However, the onset of various psychiatric disorders—such as panic disorder, posttraumatic stress, and depression—is frequently associated with a preceding period of increased environmental stress. In addition, overactivity of peripheral pituitary-adrenal function is common in patients with depression and also occurs in other psychiatric illnesses (Gold et al. 1988). Because alterations in HPA function are the most robust biological alteration found in depressed patients, recent clinical studies have focused on possible alterations in brain CRH systems associated with depression. Results indicate that increased concentrations of cerebrospinal fluid (CSF) CRH occur in some, but not all, depressed patients (Nemeroff et al. 1984). This likely reflects extrahypothalamic CRH systems, because monkey studies performed in our laboratory indicate that the CRH that accumulates in CSF has its origin in brain sites outside the hypothalamus (Kalin et al. 1987b). In addition, postmortem studies of brains collected from suicide victims reveal a decrease in the number of CRH receptors in the frontal cortex (Nemeroff et al. 1988). Although suggestive, these data, obtained from clinical research, do not directly implicate CRH systems in mediating the behavioral changes associated with depression or other states characterized by a persistence of maladaptive behaviors.

Animal studies are valuable because they allow direct manipulation of CRH systems. Data from our studies support the hypothesis that brain CRH systems mediate behaviors expressed during stressful or anxiety-provoking situations. In our studies with rats and infant

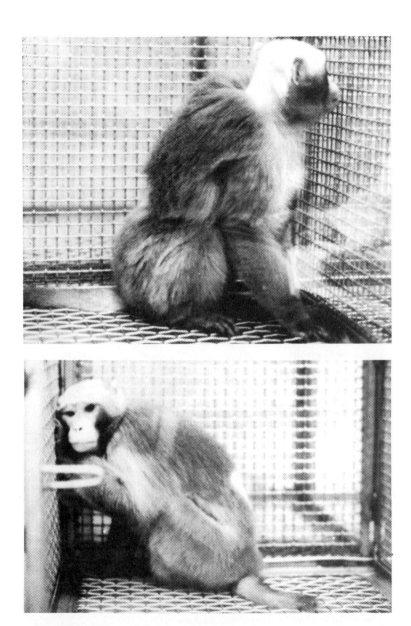

Figure 2-6. Effects of vehicle (*top*) compared with 180 μg intracerebro-ventricular-administered corticotropin-releasing hormone (CRH) (*bottom*) in adult male rhesus monkey. CRH results in huddled posture.

monkeys, we found that administration of CRH enhanced and administration of the CRH antagonist reduced stress-related behaviors. Our studies also suggest that if the "tone" of the CRH system is altered by an increase or a reduction in its activity, maladaptive or abnormal behaviors may emerge. For example, rats tested in the large arena, after receiving CRH, behaved as if they perceived the environment as a greater threat than did animals administered vehicle. In contrast, rats treated with the CRH antagonist acted boldly in the open field and even ignored important olfactory cues from conspecifics signifying danger. Studies in the infant monkeys revealed that CRH administration increased behavioral inhibition and had effects opposite of antianxiety compounds. In human children, extreme behavioral inhibition has been associated with shyness (Kagan et al. 1988), and we have suggested that behavioral inhibition in the infant monkey may be a model of human shyness (Kalin and Shelton 1989). In our studies with adult monkeys, we examined the effects of large doses of CRH and found that these doses resulted in behaviors associated with depression.

Our data suggest that increases in CRH function may in part underlie disorders associated with heightened fearfulness and withdrawal behaviors. Such syndromes might include separation anxiety, school phobia, generalized anxiety, panic and phobic disorders, social phobias, avoidant personality, extreme shyness, and depression. In contrast, reductions in CRH activity may be associated with illnesses characterized by disinhibition. These might include attention-deficit hyperactivity disorder, impulse-control disorders, and mania.

Since CRH neurons and receptors exist throughout the brain (De Souza 1987), it is interesting to speculate which CRH systems may be involved in the expression of psychopathology. Evidence from various sources suggests that CRH systems modulate the firing of noradrenergic neurons originating in the locus coeruleus (Valentino and Foote 1987; Valentino et al. 1983). This is particularly interesting because the locus coeruleus contains most of the brain's noradrenergic cell bodies and functions to regulate behavioral arousal (Cooper et al. 1982). In addition, dysregulation of the locus coeruleus has been suggested as a mechanism underlying depression and anxiety (Gold et al. 1988; Redmond 1987). Therefore, alterations in CRH systems in the region of the locus coeruleus could have an important impact on noradrenergic activity mediating states of heightened arousal associated with depression and anxiety.

REFERENCES

Aldenhoff JB, Gruol DL, Rivier J, et al: Corticotropin-releasing factor decreases postburst hyperpolarizations and excites hippocampal neurons. Science 221:875–877, 1983

Antoni FA, Palkovits M, Makara GB, et al: Immunoreactive corticotropin-releasing hormone in the hypothalamoinfundibular tract. Neuroendocrinology 36:415–423, 1983

Berridge CW, Dunn AJ: Corticotropin-releasing factor elicits naloxone sensitive stress-like alterations in exploratory behavior in mice. Regul Peptides 16:83–93, 1986

Bloom FE, Battenberg ELF, Rivier J, et al: Corticotropin-releasing factor (CRF): immunoreactive neurones and fibers in rat hypothalamus. Regul Peptides 4:43–48, 1982

Britton DR, Koob GF, Rivier J, et al: Intraventricular corticotropin-releasing factor enhances behavioral effects of novelty. Life Sci 31:363–367, 1982

Brown MR, Fisher LA: Central nervous system effects of corticotropin-releasing hormone in the dog. Brain Res 280:75–80, 1983

Brown MR, Fisher LA, Rivier J, et al: Corticotropin-releasing factor: effects on the sympathetic nervous system and oxygen consumption. Life Sci 30:207–210, 1982

Brown MR, Fisher LA, Webb V, et al: Corticotropin-releasing factor: a physiological regulator of adrenal epinephrine secretion. Brain Res 328:355–357, 1985

Bugnon CD, Fellman D, Gouget A, et al: Corticoliberin in rat brain: immunocytochemical identification and localization of a novel neuroglandular system. Neurosci Lett 30:25–30, 1982

Cooper JR, Bloom FE, Roth RH: The Biochemical Basis of Neuropharmacology, 4th Edition. New York, Oxford University Press, 1982

Cummings S, Elde R, Ells J, et al: Corticotropin-releasing factor immunoreactivity is widely distributed within the central nervous system of the rat: an immunohistochemical study. J Neurosci 3:1355–1368, 1983

De Souza EB: Corticotropin-releasing factor receptors in the rat central nervous system: characterization and regional distribution. J Neurosci 7:88–100, 1987

De Souza EB, Perrin MH, Insel TR, et al: Corticotropin-releasing factor receptors in rat forebrain: autoradiographic identification. Science 224:1449–1451, 1984

De Souza EB, Insel TR, Perrin MH, et al: Corticotropin-releasing factor receptors are widely distributed within the rat central nervous system: an autoradiographic study. J Neurosci 5:3189–3203, 1985

Ehlers CL, Henriksen SJ, Wang M, et al: Corticotropin-releasing factor produces increases in brain excitability and convulsive seizures in rats. Brain Res 278:332–336, 1983

Fischman AJ, Muldow RL: Extrahypothalamic distribution of CRF-like immunoreactivity in the rat brain. Peptides 1:149–153, 1982

Fisher LA, Rivier J, Rivier C, et al: Corticotropin-releasing factor (CRF): central effects on mean arterial pressure and heart rate in rats. Endocrinology 110:2222–2224, 1982

Gold PW, Goodwin FK, Chrousos GP: Clinical and biochemical manifestations of depression. N Engl J Med 319:413–420, 1988

Gunnar MR, Gonzalez CA, Goodlin BL, et al: Behavioral and pituitary-adrenal responses during a prolonged separation period in infant rhesus macaques. Psychoneuroendocrinology 6:65–75, 1981

Harlow HF, Suomi SJ: Induced depression in monkeys. Behav Biol 12:273–296, 1974

Kagan J, Reznick JS, Snidman N: Biological bases of childhood shyness. Science 240:167–171, 1988

Kalin NH, Carnes M: Biological correlates of attachment bond disruption in human and nonhuman primates. Prog Neuropsychopharmacol Biol Psychiatry 8:459–469, 1984

Kalin NH, Shelton SE: Defensive behaviors in infant rhesus monkeys: environmental cues and neurochemical regulation. Science 243:1718–1721, 1989

Kalin NH, Takahashi LK: Fear-motivated behavior induced by prior shock experience is mediated by corticotropin-releasing hormone systems. Brain Res 509:80–84, 1990

Kalin NH, Shelton SE, Kraemer GW, et al: Associated endocrine, physiological and behavioral changes in rhesus monkeys after intravenous CRF administration. Peptides 4:211–215, 1983a

Kalin NH, Shelton SE, Kraemer GW, et al: Corticotropin-releasing factor administered intraventricularly to rhesus monkeys. Peptides 4:217–220, 1983b

Kalin NH, Shelton SE, Barksdale CM: Separation distress in infant rhesus monkeys: effects of diazepam and Ro 15-1788. Brain Res 408:192–198, 1987a

Kalin NH, Shelton SE, Barksdale CM, et al: A diurnal rhythm in cerebrospinal fluid-corticotropin-releasing hormone different from the rhythm of pituitary adrenal activity. Brain Res 426:385–391, 1987b

Kalin NH, Shelton SE, Barksdale CM: Opiate modulation of separation-induced distress in non-human primates. Brain Res 440:285–292, 1988a

Kalin NH, Sherman JE, Takahashi LK: Antagonism of endogenous CRH systems attenuates stress-induced freezing behavior in rats. Brain Res 457:130–135, 1988b

Kalin NH, Shelton SE, Barksdale CM: Behavioral and physiological effects of CRH administered to infant primates undergoing maternal separation. Neuropsychopharmacology 2:97–104, 1989

Koob GF, Bloom FE: Corticotropin-releasing factor and behavior. Fed Proc 44:259–263, 1985

Liposits Z, Lengvari I, Vigh S, et al: Immunohistological detection of degenerating CRF-immunoreactive nerve fibers in the median eminence after lesion of paraventricular nucleus of the rat: a light and electron microscopic study. Peptides 4:941–953, 1983

McKinney WT: Biobehavioral models of depression in monkeys, in Animal Models in Psychiatry and Neurology. Edited by Hanin I, Usdin E. New York, Pergamon, 1977, pp 117–126

Merchenthaler I, Vigh S, Petrusz P, et al: The paraventricular infundibular corticotropin-releasing factor (CRF) pathway as revealed by immunocytochemistry in long-term hypophysectomized or adrenalectomized rats. Regul Peptides 5:295–306, 1983

Nemeroff CB, Wilderlov E, Bisette G, et al: Elevated concentrations of CSF corticotropin-releasing factor-like immunoreactivity in depressed patients. Science 226:1342–1344, 1984

Nemeroff CB, Owens MJ, Bissette G, et al: Reduced CRF binding sites in the frontal cortex of suicide victims. Arch Gen Psychiatry 45:577–579, 1988

Olschowka JA, O'Donohue TL, Mueller GP, et al: The distribution of corticotropin-releasing factor-like immunoreactive neurons in rat brain. Peptides 3:995–1015, 1982a

Olschowka JA, O'Donohue TL, Mueller GP, et al: Hypothalamic and extrahypothalamic distribution of CRF-like immunoreactive neurons in the rat brain. Neuroendocrinology 35:305–308, 1982b

Redmond DE: Studies of the nucleus locus coeruleus in monkeys and hypotheses for neuropsychopharmacology, in Psychopharmacology: The Third Generation of Progress. Edited by Meltzer HY. New York, Raven, 1987, pp 967–973

Reite M, Short RA: Nocturnal sleep in separated monkey infants. Arch Gen Psychiatry 35:1247–1253, 1978

Sherman JE, Kalin NH: ICV-CRH alters stress-induced freezing behavior without affecting pain sensitivity. Pharm Biochem Behav 30:801–807, 1988

Smith MA, Bissette G, Slotkin TA, et al: Release of corticotropin-releasing factor from rat brain regions in vitro. Endocrinology 118:1997–2001, 1986

Spiess J, Rivier J, Rivier C, et al: Primary structure of corticotropin-releasing factor from ovine hypothalamus. Proc Natl Acad Sci USA 78:6417–6521, 1981

Sutton RE, Koob GF, LeMoal M, et al: Corticotropin-releasing factor produces behavioral activation in rats. Nature (London) 297:331–333, 1982

Swanson LW, Sawchenko PE, Rivier J, et al: Organization of ovine corticotropin-releasing factor immunoreactive cells and fibers in the rat brain: an immunohistochemical study. Neuroendocrinology 36:165–186, 1983

Takahashi LK, Kalin NH: Role of corticotropin-releasing factor in mediating the expression of defensive behavior, in Ethoexperimental Approaches to the Study of Behavior. Edited by Blanchard RJ, Brain PF, Blanchard DC, et al. Dordrecht, Holland, Kluwer, 1989, pp 580–594

Takahashi LK, Kalin NH, Vanden Burgt JA, et al: Corticotropin-releasing factor modulates defensive-withdrawal and exploratory behavior in rats. Behav Neurosci 103:648–654, 1989

Takahashi LK, Kalin NH, Baker EW: Corticotropin-releasing factor antagonist attenuates defensive-withdrawal behavior elicited by odors of stressed conspecifics. Behav Neurosci 104:386–389, 1990

Vale W, Spiess J, Rivier C, et al: Characterization of a 41-residue ovine hypothalamic peptide that stimulates secretion of corticotropin and β-endorphin. Science 213:1394–1397, 1981

Valentino R, Foote S: Corticotropin-releasing factor disrupts sensory responses of brain noradrenergic neurons. Neuroendocrinology 45:28–36, 1987

Valentino RJ, Foote SL, Aston-Jones G: Corticotropin-releasing factor activates noradrenergic neurons of the locus coeruleus. Brain Res 270:363–367, 1983

Chapter 3

Corticotropin-Releasing Factor: Brain and Cerebrospinal Fluid Studies

**M. Adriana Vargas, M.D., Michael J. Owens, Ph.D.,
Charles B. Nemeroff, M.D., Ph.D.**

C orticotropin-releasing factor (CRF), a 41–amino acid peptide, was first isolated, sequenced, and characterized by Vale et al. (1981) from ovine hypothalami. It is the major physiological regulator of proopiomelanocortin (POMC)-derived peptide release from the pituitary gland (Rivier et al. 1982). Immunohistochemical and radioimmunoassay methods have demonstrated a heterogeneous distribution of CRF in the mammalian central nervous system (CNS) (Swanson et al. 1983). Similarly, with the use of autoradiographic and biochemical studies, high-affinity CRF binding sites, putative receptors, have been identified in the CNS (De Souza et al. 1985; Millan et al. 1986).

The most widely recognized group of CRF neurons is located in the paraventricular nucleus of the hypothalamus, which projects to the median eminence, the site of the primary plexus of the hypothalamo-hypophysial portal system (Antoni et al. 1983; Olschowka et al. 1982). Extrahypothalamic populations of CRF cell bodies have been described in association with central autonomic nuclei, the locus coeruleus, and numerous limbic and cortical areas (Bloom et al. 1982; Olschowka et al. 1982). Among the limbic areas, CRF immunoreactivity has been demonstrated in the amygdala (Fellmann et al. 1982; Merchenthaler 1984; Moga and Gray 1985), the bed nucleus of the stria terminalis, the substantia innominata, and the septum. Corticotropin-releasing factors containing nerve terminals are associated

This work was supported by NIMH Grants MH-42088, MH-40524, and MH-40159. We are grateful to Shelia Walker and Sharon Rhoden for the preparation of the manuscript.

73

with the locus coeruleus and raphe nuclei, the major cell body regions for noradrenergic and serotonergic projections, respectively.

Potassium-induced, calcium-dependent release of CRF from slices of hypothalamus, amygdala, midbrain, striatum, and cortex, similar to that of other neurotransmitters, has been demonstrated (Owens et al. 1987; Smith et al. 1986; Suda et al. 1985). These studies strongly suggest allowing CRF to fulfill the requisite criteria for consideration as a neurotransmitter in the CNS. Preclinical studies strongly suggest that CRF is involved in the centrally mediated endocrine, autonomic, and behavioral response to stress.

The effect of CRF in activating extrahypothalamic CNS neurons has been demonstrated in numerous studies. Electroencephalographic changes concordant with increased excitability in the hippocampus and cortex after intraventricular CRF administration have been observed (Ehlers et al. 1983; Marrosu et al. 1987). Several studies have also demonstrated that CRF acting in different brain regions increases sympathetic outflow and may be intimately involved in autonomic aspects of the stress response. Particularly important are the studies of Valentino and Foote (1987) and Valentino et al. (1983), which demonstrated that direct microapplication or intracisternal administration of CRF alters the firing rate of neurons in several CNS regions, including the locus coeruleus (the A_6 noradrenergic cell group), which projects throughout the CNS (Foote et al. 1983). Because the locus coeruleus contains both CRF immunoreactivity, presumably in terminals, and the A_6 noradrenergic cell bodies (Cummings et al. 1983; Swanson et al. 1983), CRF could be involved in the coordination of the autonomic and behavioral aspects of the stress response through changes in central noradrenergic activity. Chappell et al. (1986) showed that stress produces increases in CRF concentrations in the locus coeruleus and, in concert with the aforementioned electrophysiological data, might be expected to increase noradrenergic activity in the CNS.

Chappell et al. (1986) measured the concentration of CRF-like immunoreactivity in 36 microdissected rat brain areas after exposure to acute or chronic stress. Both acute and chronic stress produced changes in CRF concentrations in several brain areas.

A 50% decrease of CRF was observed in the median eminence, in both acute- and chronic-stress groups. This was associated with elevated plasma corticosterone concentrations. The decreased CRF concentration in the median eminence is thought to represent stress enhanced release of CRF from the nerve terminals into the hypothalamic-hypophysial portal circulation, which activates the hypothalamo-pituitary-adrenal (HPA) axis. Chronic and acute stress increased CRF concentrations twofold in the locus coeruleus. Chronic stress decreased the concentration of CRF in the dorsal vagal complex, whereas CRF concentrations were increased in the anterior and periventricular hypothalamic areas. All of these brain areas have been previously associated with the stress response. The decreased CRF concentration in the dorsal vagal complex is concordant with a role for CRF in regulation of the autonomic nervous system. As mentioned before, the increased CRF concentrations in the locus coeruleus are particularly interesting because CRF increases neuronal firing rates in this region, which projects throughout the brain with potentially global CNS effects. With the use of a foot-shock stress paradigm, N. Kalin (unpublished observations, 1989) confirmed the stress-induced increase in locus coeruleus CRF concentrations. In agreement with this hypothesis, Dunn and Berridge (1987) reported that CRF increases noradrenergic turnover. These findings have been confirmed after intra-locus coeruleus injection of the peptide (Butler et al., in press). Because a dysregulation of central norepinephrine containing neurons has been posited to occur in both depressive and anxiety disorders (Redmond and Huang 1979; Simson et al. 1986a, 1986b; Svensson 1987), the aforementioned findings have potentially important clinical applications.

Many behavioral and physiological changes after direct administration of CRF into the CNS have been described and support the hypothesis that central CRF may mediate the stress response (Brown 1986; Brown and Fisher 1983; Brown et al. 1982; Fisher et al. 1982, 1983). These effects are remarkably similar to those observed during the initial phase of the alarm reaction as described by Selye (1936). They are not mediated by activation of the HPA axis, however, and are insensitive to the glucocorticoid feedback (K. Britton et al. 1986a; D. Britton et al. 1986).

Central administration of CRF produces a profile of behavioral activation similar to that observed in stressed animals. Moreover, CRF also increases laboratory animals' sensitivity to stressful stimuli. Intracerebroventricular administration of CRF to rats in a familiar, nonstressful environment produces behaviors associated with increased arousal (K. Britton et al. 1986a; D. Britton et al. 1986; Koob and Bloom 1985; Sutton et al. 1982; Tazi et al. 1987a). In contrast, peripheral administration of CRF is without effect (D. Britton et al. 1986; Sutton et al. 1982). Corticotropin-releasing factor also increases the frequency of stress-induced fighting induced by mild electric foot shock, an effect that was decreased by the CRF receptor antagonist (Tazi et al. 1987b).

Other changes after central administration of CRF to laboratory animals include reduced food consumption (D. Britton et al. 1982; Gosnell et al. 1983; Levine et al. 1983; Morley and Levine 1982), diminished sexual behavior (Sirinathsinghji 1985, 1987; Sirinathsinghji et al. 1983), and alterations in locomotor activity (Koob and Bloom 1985). Many of these effects of CRF are reminiscent of the signs and symptoms of depression and anxiety disorders (DSM-III-R; American Psychiatric Association 1987). Conversely, central administration of a CRF receptor antagonist attenuates stress-induced increases in autonomic function (Brown et al. 1986), reverses stress-induced secretion of luteinizing hormone in castrated male rats (Rivier et al. 1986), and partially blocks stress-induced decreases in food consumption in food-deprived rats (Krahn et al. 1986). K. Britton et al. (1986b) also demonstrated that the CRF receptor antagonist blocks the activating and anxiogenic actions of CRF in the rat. These findings, taken together, support the hypothesis that endogenous CRF plays a preeminent role in coordinating CNS responses to stress.

Owens et al. (1989) tested the hypothesis that the therapeutic effects of antidepressant and/or anxiolytic drugs may be caused, in part, by an interaction with CRF neurons. We studied the effects of two triazolobenzodiazepines, alprazolam and adinazolam, compounds that not only possess anxiolytic effects but also purport antidepressant properties (Amsterdam et al. 1986a; Feighner et al. 1983). Of particular interest was our finding that both triazolobenzodiazepines exerted effects on CRF concentrations opposite to those of stress. In addition, Grigoriadis et al. (1988) measured the concentration of CRF receptors after chronic administration of tricyclic antidepressants and benzodiazepines to rats. They concluded that antidepressant drugs may produce their effects in part by suppressing CRF secretion in the locus coeruleus, resulting in up-regulation of brain stem CRF binding sites. These findings support the hypothesis that CRF acting as a neurotransmitter in the CNS can simultaneously activate and coordinate endocrine, autonomic, and behavioral responses involved in the stress response. Abnormalities in stress responsiveness, long postulated to play a role in the pathogenesis of anxiety and affective disorders, may involve aberrant CRF secretion.

CORTICOTROPIN-RELEASING FACTOR CHALLENGE STUDIES

In view of the behavioral changes observed in CRF-treated laboratory animals, it is plausible to hypothesize that CRF hypersecretion from hypothalamic and extrahypothalamic neurons may contribute to the hypercortisolism and behavioral symptoms characteristic of depression and anxiety disorders and, perhaps, anorexia nervosa.

A large proportion of patients that fulfill criteria for major depression exhibit hyperactivity of the HPA axis, as demonstrated by increased basal plasma cortisol concentrations (Sachar et al. 1973), increased urinary free cortisol excretion (Carrol et al. 1976), and cortisol nonsuppression in response to the synthetic glucocorticoid dexamethasone (Carrol et al. 1981; Evans and Nemeroff 1983).

In a series of studies, several investigators (Amsterdam et al. 1987a; Gold et al. 1984, 1986; Holsboer et al. 1985, 1987; Kilts et al. 1987) observed blunted ACTH but normal plasma cortisol responses to intravenous administration of ovine CRF (OCRF) in depressed patients when compared with manic, recovered depressed, and normal subjects.

Amsterdam et al. (1987a) reported that depressed patients with melancholic features showed the most robust ACTH blunting, whereas patients separated according to the dexamethasone-suppression test results had similar ACTH and cortisol responses, suggesting that the reduced ACTH response to OCRF in depressed patients is not necessarily related to dexamethasone suppression test (DST) nonsuppression. These results have been interpreted as indicative of intact negative feedback by cortisol at the pituitary level and that the blunted ACTH response observed in depressed patients may be caused by the persistently high plasma cortisol concentrations seen in those patients. Alternatively, the reduced ACTH response to CRF may be explained by a decreased density (down-regulation) of CRF receptors on the corticotroph cells and a subsequent diminished responsiveness to exogenous CRF administration. Recently, Von Bardeleben and Holsboer (1989) and R. Krishnan, C.B. Nemeroff, and B.J. Carroll (unpublished observations, 1989) noted that dexamethasone pretreatment does not abolish CRF-induced ACTH and cortisol secretion in depressed patients, as it does in healthy control subjects, providing further evidence that hypercortisolemia per se is not responsible for the blunted response to CRF in depression. In addition, Schulte et al. (1985) demonstrated that prolonged infusion (more than 24 hours) of CRF in healthy volunteers resulted in elevated ACTH and a cortisol plasma concentration resembling the pattern observed in depressed subjects. Widerlov et al. (1986) demonstrated that drug-free depressed patients had a significantly higher plasma CRF concentration than healthy control subjects. Charlton et al. (1986), however, were unable to confirm this finding.

The OCRF stimulation test has been used in other psychiatric entities related to stress, including posttraumatic stress disorder

(PTSD). Smith et al. (1989) found a blunted ACTH response to CRF in patients with PTSD only, as well as in those PTSD patients who also had major depression. Similarly, a reduced ACTH response to CRF has been observed in patients with anorexia nervosa (Hotta et al. 1986).

Some authors (Amsterdam et al. 1986b, 1988; Gold and Chrousos 1985) have suggested that in early depression there is increased ACTH and cortisol secretion in response to endogenous CRF hypersecretion. In late depression, however, continuous CRF hypersecretion produces adrenal hypertrophy and an associated increased sensitivity of the adrenal cortex to ACTH. This phenomenon might result from a prolonged exposure of the adrenal gland to small increases in circulating ACTH or related POMC-derived peptides (Amsterdam et al. 1986b; Gold et al. 1986). Increased adrenal gland size has been reported by computerized tomography in depressed patients by Amsterdam et al. (1987b), by Nemeroff et al. (1989), and in a postmortem study by Zis and Zis (1987).

These results, taken together, are compatible with the hypothesis that hyperactivity of the HPA axis in depressed patients may be caused, in part, by CRF hypersecretion at or above the hypothalamus.

CEREBROSPINAL FLUID STUDIES

In a study of pediatric patients, Hedner et al. (1989) reported higher concentrations of cerebrospinal fluid (CSF) CRF in the immediate postnatal period. Cerebrospinal fluid CRF decreased significantly during the first postnatal year compared with the immediate postnatal concentration. The adult concentration of CRF in CSF was similar to the mean concentration found in the ≥1–15 year age group. In view of the fact that CSF is one way to sample the human CNS directly, some investigators have measured CRF concentrations in CSF of psychiatric patients.

To test directly the hypothesis that CRF is hypersecreted in depressed patients, we have, in a series of studies, measured CSF CRF concentrations in drug-free psychiatric patients with several different diagnoses. In our first study (Nemeroff et al. 1984), CSF was obtained by lumbar puncture from healthy control subjects and drug-free patients with major depression, schizophrenia, or senile dementia. The depressed patients exhibited elevated CSF CRF concentrations compared with the other groups. Moreover, 11 of 23 depressed patients exhibited higher CSF CRF concentrations than the control subjects with the highest concentrations.

In a larger follow-up study of 54 drug-free depressed patients and 138 control subjects (Banki et al. 1987), the drug-free depressed patients showed, as a group, a twofold elevation in the CSF CRF concentration (Figure 3-1). We did not find a correlation between CSF CRF concentration and baseline or postdexamethasone plasma cortisol concentration. Roy et al. (1987), however, reported a significant correlation between postdexamethasone plasma cortisol concentration and CSF CRF concentration. They studied CSF CRF and plasma cortisol in 22 depressed patients and 18 healthy control subjects and found no difference in CSF CRF levels between the total group of depressed patients and the control group. The depressed patients who were DST nonsuppressors, however, showed a significantly higher CSF CRF concentration than the DST suppressors. In addition, the CSF CRF concentrations were directly correlated with 4 P.M. postdexamethasone plasma cortisol levels. These findings are similar to those reported by Davis et al. (1984), who did not find any difference between CSF CRF concentration in a small sample of depressed patients and that in control subjects.

The observation that the DST nonsuppressors showed higher levels of CSF CRF than the DST suppressors is concordant with the finding of Kaye et al. (1987), who described a positive correlation between depression severity and CSF CRF concentrations in hypercortisolemic underweight patients with anorexia nervosa.

Discrepancies between these studies and ours (Banki et al. 1987; Nemeroff et al. 1984) are thought to be results of differences in patient population. Most other researchers studied patients with recurrent episodes and multiple drug treatments, whereas our patients were largely first-episode treatment-responsive patients.

Recently, C. Risch and N. Kalin (unpublished observations, 1989) confirmed the increased CSF CRF concentrations in drug-free depressed patients. The lack of correlation between postdexamethasone plasma cortisol concentrations and CSF CRF concentrations in our studies is probably a result of the fact that cortisol secretion is mediated by more than just CRF regulation of ACTH secretion, because other neuropeptides also appear to be involved in regulating HPA axis activity. For example, Watabe et al. (1988) showed that arginine vasopressin potentiates ACTH secretion and that it may play a physiologically important role in regulating CRF-stimulated ACTH and cortisol secretion. More important, CSF CRF concentrations probably do not reflect the CRF concentration present at the pituitary corticotroph. As we mentioned at the beginning of this chapter, CRF has been found in several extrahypothalamic areas of the CNS (Owens et al. 1987; Suda et al. 1985), but little is known about the relative contribution of these areas to lumbar CSF CRF concentrations (Banki et al. 1987).

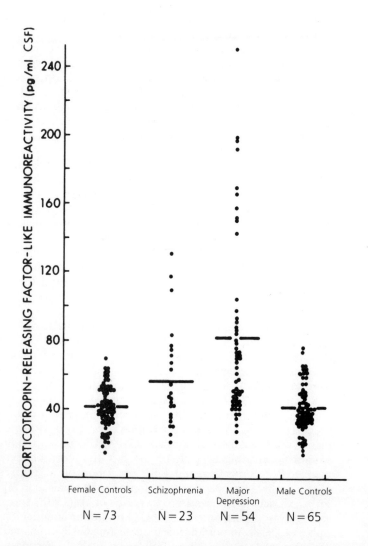

Figure 3-1. Cerebrospinal fluid (CSF) corticotropin-releasing factor-like immunoreactivity in patients with DMS-III schizophrenia, patients with DSM-III major depression, and control subjects with various peripheral neurological diseases. Reprinted from Banki CM, Bissette G, Arato M, et al: CSF corticotropin-releasing factor-like immunoreactivity in depression and schizophrenia. Am J Psychiatry 144:873–877, 1987. Copyright 1987, the American Psychiatric Association. Reprinted by permission.

For most neuropeptides found in both CSF and plasma, there is a marked plasma-CSF dissociation (Post et al. 1982), indicating that neuropeptides are secreted directly into the CSF from brain tissue and that the peptide concentrations are not derived from the general circulation (Hedner et al. 1989). Of particular interest is the study of Garrick et al. (1987), who found, in rhesus monkeys, a markedly different circadian rhythm of CSF CRF from that of plasma ACTH and cortisol as well as cortisol concentrations in the CSF (which directly reflect plasma cortisol concentrations). They demonstrated that CSF CRF exhibits peak concentrations that precede those of CSF cortisol by approximately 14 hours (almost inversely related) and that it is similarly dysynchronous with plasma ACTH and cortisol peaks.

These findings suggest that all brain CRF neurons do not act synchronously with the subset of paraventricular hypothalamic neurons believed to regulate the classical HPA axis circadian rhythm. The source of CRF in CSF and the basis for its circadian changes in concentration have not been determined (Garrick et al. 1987). Perhaps plasma CRF concentrations represent a combination of both peripheral tissue and paraventricular nucleus CRF activity and HPA axis activity, whereas CSF CRF concentrations represent extra hypothalamic CRF neurons.

Nemeroff et al. (in press) sought to determine whether increased CSF CRF concentration in depression represents a state or trait marker. Before electroconvulsive therapy (ECT), depressed patients had elevated CSF CRF concentrations. After six ECT treatments, CSF CRF concentrations were returning to normal values. These findings indicate that CSF CRF concentrations in depressed patients may represent a state, rather than a trait, marker.

The available data indicate that major depression occurs in 20–40% of patients with chronic pain (France et al. 1986; Krishnan et al. 1985a, 1985b). Some authors have considered chronic pain as a variant of depression (Blumer and Heilbroon 1982). France et al. (1988) studied whether patients with chronic pain have altered CSF CRF concentrations and whether CSF CRF concentrations in patients with chronic pain and major depression differ from those found in patients with major depression without chronic pain. Once again, we found that CSF CRF concentrations were significantly elevated in patients with major depression compared with healthy subjects. No differences were observed, however, among chronic-pain patients with major depression, those without major depression, and control subjects. Thus, patients with chronic pain who develop depression may not exhibit CRF hypersecretion.

In two other studies, we measured CSF CRF concentrations in

depressed patients, some of whom had attempted suicide, and in postmortem cisternal CSF samples from suicide victims. We observed elevated CRF concentrations in the postmortem CSF of patients who had committed suicide compared with CSF obtained from sudden-death corpses. Depressed patients as a group, however, exhibited increased CSF CRF concentrations regardless of prior suicide attempts (Arato et al. 1986, 1989).

CORTICOTROPIN-RELEASING FACTOR RECEPTORS

Considering the available data showing that depression is a major determinant of suicide (Van Praag 1986) and that more than 50% of completed suicides are accomplished by patients with major depression, we hypothesized that if CRF is chronically hypersecreted in major depression, a reduced (down-regulated) number of CRF receptors may be present in patients with depressive disorders. To test this hypothesis, we measured the number and affinity of CRF receptors in the frontal cortex of 26 suicide victims and 28 control subjects (Nemeroff et al. 1988). The suicide group exhibited a clear reduction (23%) in the number of CRF binding sites in the frontal cortex compared with control subjects (Figure 3-2). This finding further supports evidence that CRF is hypersecreted in the CNS of patients with major depression.

NEURODEGENERATIVE DISEASES

Recent studies suggest that CRF may be important in certain neurodegenerative diseases (Bissette et al. 1985; De Souza et al. 1986, 1987). Corticotropin-releasing factor concentrations are markedly reduced in the cerebral cortex of patients with Alzheimer's disease (AD) (Bissette et al. 1985; De Souza et al. 1986; Powers et al. 1987; Whitehouse et al. 1987), and some investigators have observed reduced CRF concentrations in the basal ganglia in patients with Huntington's chorea (De Souza et al. 1987). Similarly, alterations in CRF have been described in Parkinson's disease and progressive supranuclear palsy (Whitehouse et al. 1987).

Together with the aforementioned radioimmunoassay studies, several studies have shown alterations in CSF CRF concentrations in patients with AD. Mouradian et al. (1986) reported a 16% reduction of CSF CRF concentrations, and May et al. (1987) observed a 30% reduction in the CSF concentration of CRF in patients with AD. Pomara et al. (1989) did not find significant alterations in CSF CRF concentration in a relatively small group of both mild and moderately demented AD patients compared with age-matched control subjects.

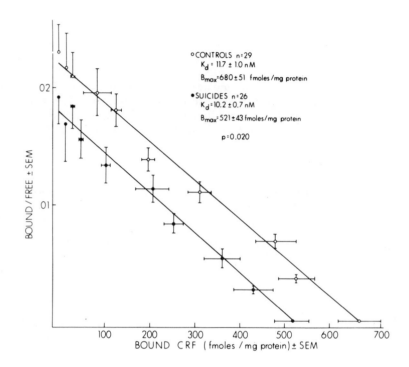

Figure 3-2. Composite Scatchard analysis using each individual frontal cortical sample. Points on composite graph represent mean ± SE for all samples from suicide victims (●) and control subjects (○). Composite Scatchard analysis was drawn graphically with maximal amount of bound ^{125}I-Tyr^0-ovine corticotropin-releasing factor (B_{max}) as determined from mean of all samples. Slope of line was determined as equal to -1/mean K_d. Hill coefficients for both groups were 1.00 ± .01. For control subjects, B_{max} = 680 ± 51 fmol per milligram of protein, dissociation affinity constant (K_d) = 11.7 ± 1.0 nmol/L, and $n = 29$. For suicide victims, B_{max} = 521 ± 43 fmol per milligram of protein, K_d = 10.2 ± .7 nmol/L, and $n = 26$. There was significant reduction in B_{max} in suicide victims compared with control subjects ($P = .020$). Reprinted with permission from Nemeroff CB, Owens MJ, Bissette G, et al: Reduced corticotropin-releasing factor binding sites in the frontal cortex of suicide victims. Arch Gen Psychiatry 45:577–579, 1988. Copyright 1988, American Medical Association.

There was a significant correlation, however, between CSF CRF concentration and the global neuropsychological deterioration rating in the AD group. This suggests that the amount of cognitive impairment may be related to the magnitude of the reduction in CSF CRF concentrations.

In summary, given the preclinical and clinical findings, CRF appears to be a neurotransmitter strongly implicated in the pathogenesis of depression, anxiety, and perhaps other psychiatric entities, including anorexia nervosa and several neurodegenerative diseases. These exciting findings suggest that the development of novel pharmacological treatments, such as a centrally acting CRF antagonist, may be useful in treating depression resistant to current treatment modalities.

REFERENCES

American Psychiatric Association: Diagnostic and Statistical Manual of Mental Disorders, 3rd Edition, Revised. Washington, DC, American Psychiatric Association, 1987

Amsterdam JD, Kaplan M, Potter L, et al: Adinazolam, a new triazolobenzodiazepine, and imipramine in the treatment of major depressive disorder. Psychopharmacology 88:484–488, 1986a

Amsterdam JD, Maislin G, Abelman E, et al: Adrenocortical responsiveness to the ACTH stimulation test in depressed patients and healthy volunteers. J Affective Disord 11:265–274, 1986b

Amsterdam JD, Maislin G, Winokur A, et al: Pituitary and adrenocortical responses to the ovine corticotropin-releasing hormone in depressed patients and healthy volunteers. Arch Gen Psychiatry 44:775–781, 1987a

Amsterdam JD, Marinelli D, Arger P, et al: Assessment of adrenal gland volume by computed tomography in depressed patients and healthy volunteers. Psychiatry Res 21:189–197, 1987b

Amsterdam JD, Maislin G, Winokur A, et al: The oCRF stimulation test before and after clinical recovery from depression. J Affective Disord 14:213–222, 1988

Antoni FA, Palkovits M, Makara GB, et al: Immunoreactive corticotropin releasing hormone in the hypothalamoinfundibular tract. Neuroendocrinology 36:415–423, 1983

Arato M, Banki CM, Nemeroff CB, et al: Hypothalamic-pituitary-adrenal axis in suicide. Ann NY Acad Sci 487:263–270, 1986

Arato M, Banki CM, Bissette G, et al: Elevated CSF CRF in suicide victims. Biol Psychiatry 25:355–359, 1989

Banki CM, Bissette G, Arato M, et al: CSF corticotropin-releasing factor-like immunoreactivity in depression and schizophrenia. Am J Psychiatry 144:873–877, 1987

Bissette G, Reynolds GP, Kilts CD, et al: Corticotropin-releasing factor-like immunoreactivity in senile dementia of the Alzheimer type. J Am Med Assoc 254:3067–3069, 1985

Bloom RE, Battenberg ELF, Rivier J, et al: Corticotropin-releasing factor (CRF) immunoreactive neurons and fibers in rat hypothalamus. Regul Peptides 4:43–48, 1982

Blumer D, Heilbroon M: Chronic pain as a variant of depressive disease: the pain prone disorder. J Nerv Ment Dis 170:381–406, 1982

Britton DR, Koob GF, Rivier J, et al: Intraventricular corticotropin releasing factor enhances behavioral effects of novelty. Life Sci 31:363–367, 1982

Britton DR, Varela M, Garcia A, et al: Dexamethasone suppresses pituitary-adrenal but not behavioral effects of centrally administered CRF. Life Sci 38:211–216, 1986

Britton KT, Lee G, Dana R, et al: Activating and "anxiogenic" effects of corticotropin releasing factor are not inhibited by blockade of the pituitary-adrenal system with dexamethasone. Life Sci 39:1281–1286, 1986a

Britton KT, Lee G, Vale W, et al: Corticotropin releasing factor (CRF) receptor antagonist blocks activating and anxiogenic actions of CRF in rat. Brain Res 369:303–306, 1986b

Brown M: Corticotropin-releasing factor: central nervous system sites of action. Brain Res 399:10–14, 1986

Brown MR, Fisher LA: Central nervous system effects of corticotropin releasing factor in the dog. Brain Res 280:75–79, 1983

Brown MR, Fisher LA, Siess J, et al: Corticotropin-releasing factor: actions on the sympathetic nervous system and metabolism. Endocrinology 111:928–931, 1982

Brown MR, Gray TS, Fisher LA: Corticotropin-releasing factor receptor antagonist: effects on the autonomic nervous system and cardiovascular function. Regul Peptides 16:321–329, 1986

Butler PD, Weiss JM, Stout JC, et al: Corticotropin-releasing factor produces fear-enhancing and behavioral activating effects following infusion into the locus coeruleus. J Neurosci (in press)

Carrol BJ, Curtis GC, Davies BM, et al: Urinary free cortisol excretion in depression. Psychol Med 6:43–50, 1976

Carrol BJ, Feinberg M, Greden JF, et al: A specific laboratory test for the diagnosis of melancholia. Arch Gen Psychiatry 38:15–22, 1981

Chappell PB, Smith MA, Kilts CD, et al: Alterations in corticotropin releasing factor-like immunoreactivity in discrete rat brain regions after acute and chronic stress. J Neurosci 6:2908–2914, 1986

Charlton BG, Leake A, Ferrier IN, et al: Corticotropin-releasing factor in plasma of depressed patients and controls. Lancet 1:161–162, 1986

Cummings S, Elde R, Ells J, et al: Corticotropin-releasing factor immuno-reactivity is widely distributed within the central nervous system of the rat: an immunohistochemical study. J Neurosci 3:1355–1368, 1983

Davis K, Davis B, Mohs R, et al: CSF corticotropin-releasing factor in neuropsychiatric diseases. Paper presented at the annual meeting of the American Psychiatric Association, Washington, DC, May 1984

De Souza EB, Insel TR, Perrin MH, et al: Corticotropin-releasing factor receptors are widely distributed within the rat central nervous system: an autoradiographic study. J Neurosci 5:3189–3203, 1985

De Souza EB, Whitehouse PJ, Kuhar MJ, et al: Reciprocal changes in corticotropin-releasing factor (CRF)-like immunoreactivity and CRF receptors in cerebral cortex of Alzheimer's disease. Nature 319:593–595, 1986

De Souza EB, Whitehouse PJ, Folstein SE, et al: Corticotropin-releasing hormone (CRH) is decreased in the basal ganglia in Huntington's disease. Brain Res 437:355–359, 1987

Dunn AJ, Berridge CW: Corticotropin-releasing factor administration elicits a stress-like activation of cerebral catecholaminergic systems. Pharmacol Biochem Behav 27:685–691, 1987

Ehlers CL, Henriksen SJ, Wang M, et al: Corticotropin-releasing factor produces increases in brain excitability and convulsive seizures in rats. Brain Res 278:332–336, 1983

Evans DL, Nemeroff CB: Use of dexamethasone suppression test using DSM III criteria on an inpatient psychiatric unit. Biol Psychiatry 18:505–511, 1983

Feighner JP, Aden GC, Fabre LF, et al: Comparison of alprazolam, im-ipramine, and placebo in the treatment of depression. J Am Med Assoc 249:3057–3064, 1983

Fellmann D, Bugnon C, Gouget A: Immunocytochemical demonstration of corticoliberin-like immunoreactivity (CLI) in neurons of the rat amyg-dala central nucleus (ACN). Neurosci Lett 34:253–258, 1982

Fisher LA, Rivier J, Rivier C, et al: Corticotropin releasing factor (CRF):

central effects on mean arterial pressure and heart rate in rats. Endocrinology 110:2222–2224, 1982

Fisher LA, Jessen G, Brown MR: Corticotropin-releasing factor (CRF) mechanism to elevate mean anterial pressure and heart rate. Regul Peptides 5:153–161, 1983

Foote SL, Bloom FE, Aston-Jones G: Nucleus locus coeruleus: new evidence of anatomical and physiological specificity. Physiol Rev 63:844–914, 1983

France RD, Houpt JL, Skott A, et al: Depression as a psychopathological disorder in chronic low back pain patients. J Psychosom Res 30:127–133, 1986

France RD, Urban B, Krishnan KRR, et al: CSF corticotropin-releasing factor-like immunoreactivity in chronic pain patients with and without major depression. Biol Psychiatry 23:86–88, 1988

Garrick NA, Hill JL, Szele FG, et al: Corticotropin-releasing factor: a marked circadian rhythm in primate cerebrospinal fluid peaks in the evening and is inversely related to the cortisol circadian rhythm. Endocrinology 121:1329–1334, 1987

Gold PW, Chrousos GP: Clinical studies with corticotropin-releasing factor: implications for the diagnosis and pathophysiology of depression, Cushing's disease and adrenal insufficiency. Psychoneuroendocrinology 10:401–419, 1985

Gold PW, Chrousos G, Kellner C, et al: Psychiatric implications of basic and clinical studies with corticotropin-releasing factor. Am J Psychiatry 141:619–627, 1984

Gold PW, Loriaux DL, Roy A, et al: Responses to corticotropin-releasing hormone in the hypercortisolism of depression and Cushing's disease. N Engl J Med 314:1329–1335, 1986

Gosnell BA, Morley JE, Levine AS: A comparison of the effects of corticotropin-releasing factor and sauvagine on food intake. Pharmacol Biochem Behav 19:771–775, 1983

Grigoriadis DE, Pearsall D, De Souza EB: Effects of chronic antidepressant and benzodiazepine treatment on corticotropin-releasing factor receptors in rat brain and pituitary. Neuropsychopharmacology 2:53–60, 1988

Hedner J, Hedner T, Lundell KH, et al: Cerebrospinal fluid concentrations of neurotensin and corticotropin-releasing factor in pediatric patients. Biol Neonate 55:260–267, 1989

Holsboer F, Bardeleben U, Green A, et al: Blunted corticotropin-releasing factor in depression. N Engl J Med 311:1127, 1985

Holsboer F, Gerken A, Stalla GK, et al: Blunted aldosterone and ACTH release after human CRF administration in depressed patients. Am J Psychiatry 144:229–231, 1987

Hotta M, Shibasaki T, Masuda A, et al: The responses of plasma adrenocorticotropin and cortisol to corticotropin-releasing hormone (CRH) and cerebrospinal fluid immunoreactive CRH in anorexia nervosa patients. J Clin Endocrinol Metab 62:319–324, 1986

Kaye WH, Gwirtsman HE, George DT, et al: Elevated cerebrospinal fluid levels of immunoreactive corticotropin-releasing hormone in anorexia nervosa: relation to state of nutrition, adrenal function and intensity of depression. J Clin Endocrinol Metab 64:203–208, 1987

Kilts CD, Bissette G, Krishnan KRR, et al: The preclinical and clinical neurobiology of corticotropin-releasing factor (CRF), in Hormones and Depression. Edited by Halbreich U, Rose RM. New York, Raven, 1987, pp 297–312

Koob GF, Bloom FE: Corticotropin-releasing factor and behavior. Fed Am Soc Exp Biol 44:259–263, 1985

Krahn DD, Gosnell BA, Grace M, et al: CRF antagonist partially reverses CRF- and stress-induced effects on feeding. Brain Res Bull 17:285–289, 1986

Krishnan KRR, France RD, Pelton S, et al: Chronic pain and depression I: classification of depression in chronic low back pain patients. Pain 22:279–287, 1985a

Krishnan KRR, France RD, Pelton S, et al: Chronic pain and depression II: symptoms of anxiety in chronic low back pain patients and their relationship to subtypes of depression. Pain 22:289–294, 1985b

Levine AS, Rogers B, Kneip J, et al: Effect of centrally administered corticotropin-releasing factor (CRF) on multiple feeding paradigms. Neuropharmacology 22:337–339, 1983

Marrosu F, Mereu G, Fratta W, et al: Different epileptogenic activities of murine and ovine corticotropin-releasing factor. Brain Res 408:394–398, 1987

May C, Rapoport SI, Tomai TP, et al: Cerebrospinal fluid concentrations of corticotropin-releasing hormone (CRH) and corticotropin (ACTH) are reduced in patients with Alzheimer's disease. Neurology 37:535–538, 1987

Merchenthaler I: Corticotropin releasing factor (CRF)-like immunoreactivity in the rat central nervous system: extrahypothalamic distribution. Peptides 5:53–69, 1984

Millan MA, Jacobowitz DM, Hauger RL, et al: Distribution of corticotropin-releasing factor receptors in primate brain. Proc Natl Acad Sci USA 83:1921–1925, 1986

Moga MM, Gray TS: Evidence for corticotropin-releasing factor, neurotensin and somatostatin in the neural pathway from the central nucleus of the amygdala to the parabrachial nucleus. J Comp Neurol 241:275–284, 1985

Morley JE, Levine AS: Corticotropin releasing factor, grooming and ingestive behavior. Life Sci 31:1459–1464, 1982

Mouradian MM, Farah JM, Mohre E, et al: Spinal fluid CRF reduction in Alzheimer's disease. Neuropeptides 8:393–400, 1986

Nemeroff CB, Widerlov E, Bissette G, et al: Elevated concentrations of CSF corticotropin-releasing factor-like immunoreactivity in depressed patients. Science 226:1342–1344, 1984

Nemeroff CB, Owens MJ, Bissette G, et al: Reduced corticotropin releasing factor binding sites in the frontal cortex of suicide victims. Arch Gen Psychiatry 45:577–579, 1988

Nemeroff CB, Krishnan KRR, Leder RA, et al: The adrenal gland in depressed patients: a pilot computed tomography study. Paper presented at the 27th annual meeting of the American College of Neuropsychopharmacology, 1989

Nemeroff CB, Bissette G, Akil H, et al: Cerebrospinal fluid neuropeptides in depressed patients treated with ECT: corticotropin-releasing factor, β-endorphin and somatostatin. Br J Psychiatry (in press)

Olschowka JA, O'Donohue TL, Mueller GP, et al: Hypothalamic and extrahypothalamic distribution of CRF-like immunoreactive neurons in the rat brain. Neuroendocrinology 35:305–308, 1982

Owens MJ, Maynor B, Nemeroff CB: Release of corticotropin-releasing factor (CRF) from rat prefrontal cortex in vitro. Soc Neurosci Abstr 13:1110, 1987

Owens MJ, Bissette G, Nemeroff CB: Acute effects of alprazolam and adinazolam on the concentrations of corticotropin-releasing factor in rat brain. Synapse 4:196–202, 1989

Pomara N, Singh RR, Deptula D, et al: CSF corticotropin-releasing factor (CRF) in Alzheimer's disease: its relationship to severity of dementia and mondamine metabolites. Biol Psychiatry 26:500–504, 1989

Post RM, Gold P, Rubinow DR, et al: Peptides in cerebrospinal fluid of neuropsychiatric patients: an approach to central nervous system peptide function. Life Sci 31:1–15, 1982

Powers RE, Walker LC, De Souza EB, et al: Immunohistochemical study of neurons containing corticotropin-releasing factor in Alzheimer's disease. Synapse 1:405–410, 1987

Redmond DE Jr, Huang YH: Current concept II: new evidence for a locus coeruleus-norepinephrine connection with anxiety. Life Sci 25:2149–2162, 1979

Rivier C, Brownstein M, Spiess J, et al: In vivo corticotropin-releasing factor-induced secretion of adrenocorticotropin, β-endorphin and corticosterone. Endocrinology 110:272–278, 1982

Rivier C, Rivier J, Vale W: Stress-induced inhibition of reproductive functions: role of endogenous corticotropin-releasing factor. Science 231:607–609, 1986

Roy A, Pickar D, Paul S, et al: CSF corticotropin-releasing hormone in depressed patients and normal control subjects. Am J Psychiatry 144:641–645, 1987

Sachar EJ, Hellman L, Roffwang HP, et al: Disrupted 24 hour patterns of cortisol secretion in psychotic depression. Arch Gen Psychiatry 28:19–24, 1973

Schulte HM, Chrousos GP, Gold PW, et al: Continuous administration of synthetic ovine corticotropin-releasing factor in man: physiological and pathophysiological implications. J Clin Invest 75:1781–1785, 1985

Selye H: A syndrome produced by diverse noxious agents. Nature 138:32, 1936

Simson PG, Weiss JM, Ambrose MJ, et al: Infusion of a monoamine oxidase inhibitor into the locus coeruleus can prevent stress-induced behavioral depression. Biol Psychiatry 21:724–734, 1986a

Simson PG, Weiss JM, Hoffman LJ, et al: Reversal of behavioral depression by infusion of an alpha-2-adrenergic agonist into the locus coeruleus. Neuropharmacology 25:385–389, 1986b

Sirinathsinghji DJS: Modulation of lordosis behaviour in the female rat by corticotropin releasing factor, β-endorphin and gonadotropin-releasing hormone in the mesencephalic central gray. Brain Res 336:45–55, 1985

Sirinathsinghji DJS: Inhibitory influence of corticotropin releasing factor on components of sexual behavior in the male rat. Brain Res 407:185–190, 1987

Sirinathsinghji DJS, Rees LH, Rivier J, et al: Corticotropin-releasing factor is a potent inhibitor of sexual receptivity in the female rat. Nature 305:232–235, 1983

Smith MA, Bissette G, Slotkin TA, et al: Release of corticotropin-releasing factor from rat brain regions in vitro. Endocrinology 118:1997–2001, 1986

Smith MA, Davidson J, Ritchie JC, et al: The corticotropin-releasing hormone test in patients with posttraumatic stress disorder. Biol Psychiatry 26:349–355, 1989

Suda T, Yajima F, Tomori N, et al: In vitro study of immunoreactive corticotropin releasing factor release from the rat hypothalamus. Life Sci 37:1499–1505, 1985

Sutton RE, Koob GF, LeMoal M, et al: Corticotropin releasing factor produces behavioural activation in rats. Nature 297:331–333, 1982

Svensson TH: Peripheral, autonomic regulation of locus coeruleus noradrenergic neurons in brain: putative implications for psychiatry and psychopharmacology. Psychopharmacology 92:1–7, 1987

Swanson LW, Sawchenko PE, Rivier J, et al: Organization of ovine corticotropin-releasing factor immunoreactive cells and fibers in the rat brain: an immunohistochemical study. Neuroendocrinology 36:165–186, 1983

Tazi A, Swerdlow NR, LeMoal M, et al: Behavioral activation by CRF: evidence for involvement of the ventral forebrain. Life Sci 41:41–49, 1987a

Tazi A, Dantzer R, LeMoal M, et al: Corticotropin-releasing factor antagonist blocks stress-induced fighting in rats. Regul Peptides 18:37–42, 1987b

Vale W, Spiess J, Rivier C, et al: Characterization of 41-residue ovine hypothalamic peptide that stimulates secretion of corticotropin and β-endorphin. Science 213:1394–1397, 1981

Valentino RJ, Foote SL: Corticotropin-releasing factor disrupts sensory responses of brain noradrenergic neurons. Neuroendocrinology 45:28–36, 1987

Valentino RJ, Foote SL, Aston-Jones G: Corticotropin releasing factor activates noradrenergic neurons of the locus coeruleus. Brain Res 270:363–367, 1983

Van Praag HM: Biological suicide research: outcome and limitations. Biol Psychiatry 21:1305–1323, 1986

Von Bardeleben U, Holsboer F: Cortisol response to a combined dexamethasone-human corticotropin-releasing hormone challenge in patients with depression. J Neuroendocrinology 1:485–488, 1989

Watabe T, Tanaka K, Kumagae M, et al: Role of endogenous arginine vasopressin in potentiating corticotropin-releasing hormone-stimulated corticotropin secretion in man. J Clin Endocrinol Metab 66:1132–1137, 1988

Whitehouse PJ, Vale WW, Zweig RM, et al: Reductions of corticotropin-releasing factor-like immunoreactivity in cerebral cortex in Alzheimer's disease, Parkinson's disease and progressive supranuclear palsy. Neurology 37:905–909, 1987

Widerlov E, Ekman R, Wahlestedt C: Elevated corticotropin-releasing factor-like immunoreactivity in plasma from major depressives, in Proceedings of the 15th International Congress Collegium Internationale Neuro-Psychopharmacologium. New York, Raven, 1986, p 207

Zis K, Zis A: Increased adrenal weight in victims of violent suicide. Am J Psychiatry 144:1214–1216, 1987

Chapter 4

Relationship Between Cerebrospinal Fluid Peptides and Neurotransmitters in Depression

S. Craig Risch, M.D., Richard J. Lewine, Ph.D.,
Rita D. Jewart, Ph.D., William E. Pollard, Ph.D.,
Jane M. Caudle, M.Ln., Ned H. Kalin, M.D.,
Mark Stipetic, B.S., Mary B. Eccard, R.N., M.S.,
Emile D. Risby, M.D.

Alterations in cerebrospinal fluid (CSF) catecholamines and their metabolites in the major affective disorders have been extensively reported in the literature. Significant alterations in CSF homovanillic acid (HVA), 3-methoxy-4-hydroxyphenylglycol (MHPG), and 5-hydroxyindoleacetic acid (5-HIAA)—the major central nervous system (CNS) metabolites of dopamine, norepinephrine, and serotonin, respectively—have been reported in isolated, but not all, studies of patients with affective disorders (Berger et al. 1980; Gerner et al. 1984; Gjerris et al. 1987; Koslow et al. 1983; Stahl 1985). Alterations in these CNS neurotransmitter metabolites do not appear to be generic to all affective disorders but appear to occur in specific subtypes of affective disorders (Gibbons and Davis 1986), for example, bipolar versus unipolar (Agren 1980), delusional versus nondelusional (Aberg-Wistedt et al. 1985), or melancholic versus nonmelancholic (Asberg et al. 1984; Roy et al. 1985). Furthermore, these alterations, when they occur, most commonly appear to be state dependent, occurring during depression and typically normalizing when the patient recovers and becomes euthymic (Berrettini et al. 1985; Traskman-Bendz et al. 1984).

In addition to these studies of CSF neurotransmitter metabolites in affective disorders, there is a vast literature documenting abnormalities of the hypothalamic-pituitary-adrenal (HPA) axis in patients with affective disorders. Activation of the HPA axis is reflected in glucocorticoid hypersecretion, flattened cortisol circadian periodicity, and an abnormal dexamethasone suppression test (Carroll et al. 1981; Stokes et al. 1975). Although clinical abnormalities occur at each level of the HPA axis, these abnormalities appear to be secondary to central (presumably limbic-hippocampal) dysregulation (Gold et al. 1986; Sapolsky 1989). With respect to the central dysregulation of the HPA axis in patients with affective disorders, Nemeroff et al. (1984) and Banki et al. (1987) reported elevations in CSF corticotropin-releasing factor (CRF) in depressed patients.

To date, the relationship (if any) between the neurotransmitter and neuroendocrine abnormalities is only beginning to be elucidated (Berrettini et al. 1988; Roy et al. 1985; Widerlöv et al. 1988). Our group at the Emory University School of Medicine has been studying CSF MHPG, HVA, and 5-HIAA as indices of CNS neurotransmitter activity and CSF CRF, ACTH, and 24-hour urinary free cortisol secretion as indices of limbic HPA axis regulation in patients with affective disorders and matched control subjects. In addition, we have been exploring the relationship between CNS neurotransmitter activity (as reflected in CSF MHPG, HVA, and 5-HIAA) and limbic HPA axis activity (as reflected in 24-hour urinary free cortisol and CSF ACTH and CRF). It is hypothesized that simultaneous metabolic assessments of these two systems might provide some insight into the neurochemical regulation of the limbic HPA axis in healthy volunteers. Furthermore, because dopaminergic, noradrenergic, and serotonergic mechanisms have all been implicated in the pathophysiology of limbic HPA axis dysregulation in depressed patients, this same strategy might further "dissect" or elucidate the CNS neurotransmitter pathogenesis of limbic HPA axis abnormalities in affective illness.

METHODS

All subjects were medically healthy as determined by history and physical and laboratory examinations. All subjects were not drug users as determined by history and urine toxicology screens. All subjects were medication-free for a minimum of seven days. All subjects, patients and healthy, were hospitalized at the Clinical Research Unit at the Emory University School of Medicine. At 7:30 A.M., the subjects had standard lumbar punctures for research studies. Twelve cubic centimeters of CSF was obtained from the L4-L5 interspace with the patient in the lateral decubitus position. Cerebrospinal fluid concentrations of MHPG, 5-HIAA, and HVA were determined by HPLC with electrochemical detection in S.C. Risch's laboratory. Urinary free cortisol from 24-hour urine collections was prepared by established radioimmunoassay methodology in Dr. Risch's laboratory. Cerebrospinal fluid concentrations of CRF and ACTH were determined by established radioimmunoassay methodology in N.H. Kalin's laboratory.

All subjects received a Schedule for Affective Disorders and Schizophrenia (SADS) interview (Endicott and Spitzer 1979) by an experienced clinician; subsequently, a diagnosis based on Research Diagnostic Criteria (RDC) was established and validated in a weekly consensus diagnostic meeting.

RESULTS

In this preliminary report, we describe CSF concentrations of MHPG, 5-HIAA, HVA, CRF, and ACTH as well as 24-hour urinary free cortisol secretion in 21 patients meeting RDC for major depression ($n = 16$) or bipolar depression ($n = 5$) and in 87 matched healthy control subjects. As we show in Table 4-1 and Figures 4-1 through 4-5, CSF concentrations of HVA, 5-HIAA, MHPG, ACTH, and 24-hour urinary free cortisol did not significantly differ among the subjects with major depression or bipolar depression and the healthy control group.

There was a nonsignificant trend for the depressed subjects to have higher 24-hour urinary free cortisol secretion, but this failed to reach statistical significance because of the large standard deviations of values, particularly in the depressed group. Nevertheless, as we show in Table 4-1 and Figure 4-6 and as reported by Nemeroff et al. (1984)

Table 4-1. Comparison of depressed and matched healthy subjects on five cerebrospinal fluid variables, 24-hour urinary free cortisol, and mean ventricle-to-brain ratio (VBR)

	Depressed		Healthy		
	Mean ± SE	*n*	Mean ± SE	*n*	Significance (*P*)
MHPG	44.4 ± 2.6	21	40.7 ± .8	92	.19
5-HIAA	99.4 ± 8.5	21	88.1 ± 3.8	92	.71
HVA	159.2 ± 16.4	21	157.3 ± 7.4	92	.91
ACTH	73.8 ± 7.4	20	66.2 ± 3.0	84	.29
CRF	79.9 ± 7.6	20	61.2 ± 3.8	84	.03
Cortisol	76.5 ± 20.2	14	47.6 ± 5.0	78	.19
VBR	7.6 ± .53	14	8.4 ± .22	67	.14

Note. MHPG, 3-methoxy-4-hydroxyphenylglycol; 5-HIAA, 5-hydroxyindoleacetic acid; HVA, homovanillic acid; CRF, corticotropin-releasing factor.

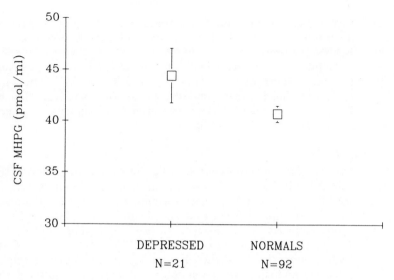

Figure 4-1. Cerebrospinal fluid 3-methoxy-4-hydroxyphenylglycol (CSF MHPG; pmol/ml) in 21 depressed patients and 92 matched healthy (normal) volunteers. Values are means ± SE.

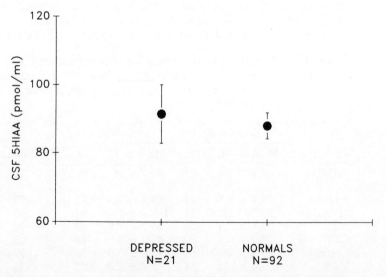

Figure 4-2. Cerebrospinal fluid 5-hydroxyindoleacetic acid (CSF 5-HIAA; pmol/ml) in 21 depressed patients and 92 matched healthy (normal) volunteers. Values are means ± SE.

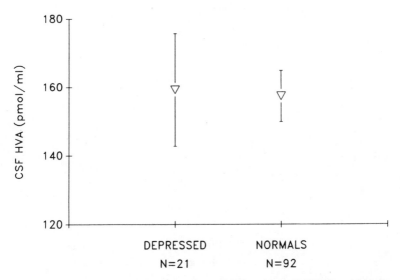

Figure 4-3. Cerebrospinal fluid homovanillic acid (CSF HVA; pmol/ml) in 21 depressed patients and 92 matched healthy (normal) volunteers. Values are means ± SE.

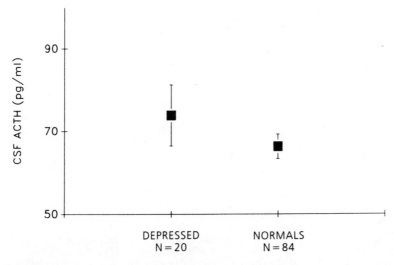

Figure 4-4. Cerebrospinal fluid (CSF) ACTH (pg/ml) in 20 depressed patients and 84 matched healthy (normal) volunteers. Values are means ± SE.

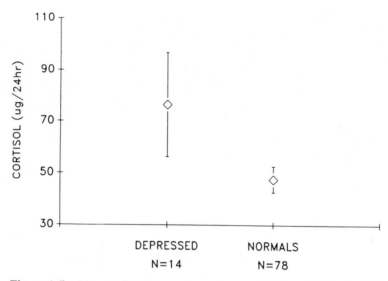

Figure 4-5. Twenty-four–hour urinary free cortisol (μg/24) in 14 depressed patients and 78 matched healthy (normal) volunteers. Values are means $\pm$ SE.

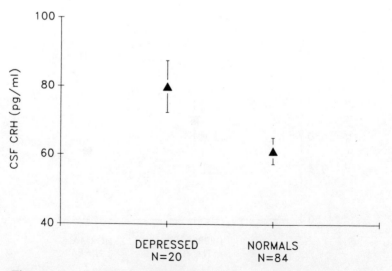

Figure 4-6. Cerebrospinal fluid corticotropin-releasing hormone (CSF CRH; pg/ml) in 20 depressed patients and 84 matched healthy (normal) volunteers. Values are means $\pm$ SE.

and Banki et al. (1987), CRF concentrations were significantly higher in the depressed group compared with the matched control subjects (depressed—79.9 ± 7.6 [mean $\pm$ SE], $n = 20$; healthy—61.2 ± 3.8, $n = 84$; $P = .034$). The differences in CSF CRF concentrations between the depressed patients and healthy subjects could not be accounted for by differences in age, sex, height, or weight between the two groups (Banki and Molinar 1981).

In the healthy subjects, 5-HIAA was significantly correlated with HVA ($r = .76$, $n = 92$, $P = .000$) and weakly correlated with MHPG ($r = .37$, $n = 92$, $P = .000$), and HVA was weakly correlated with MHPG ($r = .27$, $n = 92$, $P = .010$). Similarly, in the depressed subjects, 5-HIAA was significantly correlated with HVA ($r = .80$, $n = 21$, $P = .000$) and MHPG ($r = .74$, $n = 21$, $P = .000$), and HVA was significantly correlated with MHPG ($r = .51$, $n = 21$, $P = .02$).

In neither group were concentrations of CSF CRF or ACTH significantly correlated with concentrations of CSF 5-HIAA, HVA, or MHPG, except for a nonsignificant negative correlation between CSF CRH and CSF HVA in the depressed group ($r = -.42$, $n = 20$, $P = .07$). In both groups, CSF CRH and CSF ACTH were weakly correlated with each other (healthy—$r = .30$, $n = 84$, $P = .005$; depressed—$r = .24$, $n = 20$, $P = .30$). Twenty-four–hour urinary free cortisol did not correlate with any of the variables studied in either group.

DISCUSSION

Our data do not demonstrate any significant mean differences in CSF MHPG, 5-HIAA, or HVA between our depressed patients and our healthy volunteers. This lack of significant difference could not be attributed to any differences in age, sex, height, or weight composition among the subject groups. As we already noted, some studies have reported differences in some of these CSF neurotransmitter metabolites between depressed patients and control subjects. For example, Koslow et al. (1983) reported elevated concentrations of CSF MHPG in depressed patients compared with matched healthy control subjects. Our data suggest a nonsignificant trend toward higher CSF MHPG in our depressed subjects. Our depressed-subject population is much smaller than that of Koslow et al. (1983), so if our observed differences persist in a larger sample size, these differences would presumably reach statistical significance and be consistent with the report of Koslow et al. (1983).

Aberg-Wistedt et al. (1985) reported higher CSF concentrations of HVA and 5-HIAA in delusional depressed patients compared with nondelusional depressed patients. Asberg et al. (1984) reported lower concentrations of CSF 5-HIAA and HVA in melancholic patients compared with control subjects. Similarly, Roy et al. (1985) reported lower concentrations of HVA and other dopamine metabolites in melancholic depressed patients compared with nonmelancholic depressed patients. Agren (1980), Gibbons and Davis (1986), and others have also suggested discrete biological subtypes of depression related to specific CSF neurotransmitter profiles and patterns. Our depressed-subject group is not large enough to test these hypotheses by dividing our depressed subjects into these specific diagnostic or symptom-pattern subtypes.

Our preliminary results do, however, replicate the reports of Nemeroff et al. (1984) and Banki et al. (1987) of elevations of CSF CRF in subjects with major depression and bipolar depression compared with matched control subjects. As discussed in detail in Chapters 1 and 3, these elevations in CSF CRF in depressed patients appear to be state related and may be of profound mechanistic significance in the pathophysiology of many of the signs and symptoms of depression, including sleep, appetite, locomotor, cognitive, and memory disturbances.

Our results do not demonstrate any robust and significant correlations among CSF concentrations of CRF or ACTH or among 24-hour urinary free cortisol and CSF concentrations of MHPG, HVA, and 5-HIAA in our depressed patients or our healthy control subjects. In this regard, Widerlöv et al. (1988) reported a significant negative correlation between CSF CRF and CSF MHPG ($r = -.72$, $P = .02$) in healthy volunteers and also reported significant *positive* correlations between CSF CRF and CSF 5-HIAA ($r = .59$, $P = .004$) and between CSF CRF and CSF HVA ($r = .44$, $P = .04$) in depressed patients. In contrast, our data suggest only a low nonsignificant correlation ($r = .13$, $P = .23$) between CSF CRF and CSF MHPG in our healthy volunteers and a nonsignificant *negative* correlation between CSF CRF and CSF 5-HIAA ($r = -.11$, $P = .64$) and between CSF CRF and CSF HVA ($r = -.42$, $P = .07$). Roy et al. (1985) reported no significant correlations between CSF CRF and CSF MHPG ($r = .33$, NS), CSF HVA ($r = .18$, NS), and CSF 5-HIAA ($r = .02$, NS) in 20 depressed patients. The reasons for these discrepancies among studies may reflect small sample sizes and suggest the need for further studies.

Berrettini et al. (1988) reported significant high correlations between CSF CRF and CSF ACTH ($r = .71$, $P = .001$, $n = 16$) in healthy volunteers. Our data suggest somewhat weaker correlations between CSF CRF and CSF ACTH in healthy volunteers ($r = .30$, $P = .005$, $n = 84$) and depressed patients ($r = .24$, $P = .30$, $n = 20$).

In keeping with the report of Widerlöv et al. (1988) of no relationship of CSF CRF to either pre- or post-dexamethasone cortisol levels, we have observed no significant relationships between CSF CRF and 24-hour urinary free cortisol in our healthy volunteers ($r = .19$, $P = .11$, $n = 69$) or our depressed patients ($r = -.22$, $P = .49$, $n = 12$). Within our large healthy-subject population, 24-hour urinary free cortisol, CSF CRF and ACTH (as indices of limbic HPA activity), and CSF MHPG, 5-HIAA, and HVA (as indices of CNS neurotransmitter activity) do not seem to be robustly or significantly correlated. Thus, these results suggest that none of these three CNS neurotransmitter systems, at least as reflected cross-sectionally in their major CSF metabolite concentrations, plays a major role in the normal CNS neuroregulation of the normal limbic HPA axis.

The role of these CNS neurotransmitter systems in the dysregulation of limbic HPA activity in patients with affective disorders awaits further study. Our current sample size of depressed subjects is not large enough to meaningfully divide our depressed subjects nosologically into unipolar and bipolar groups, delusional and nondelusional groups, or melancholic and nonmelancholic groups (Standish-Barry et al. 1986). Thus, much larger groups of depressed subjects will need to be studied before differences between, or correlations within, diagnostic subtypes of patients with affective disorders in indices of CNS neurotransmitter activity and HPA axis activity can be adequately elucidated.

REFERENCES

Aberg-Wistedt A, Wistedt B, Bertilsson L: Higher CSF levels of HVA and 5-HIAA in delusional compared to nondelusional depression. Arch Gen Psychiatry 42:925–926, 1985

Agren H: Symptom patterns in unipolar and bipolar depression correlating with monoamine metabolites in the cerebrospinal fluid, I: general patterns. Psychiatry Res 3:211–223, 1980

Asberg M, Bertilsson L, Martensson B, et al: CSF monoamine metabolites in melancholia. Acta Psychiatr Scand 69:201–219, 1984

Banki CM, Molinar G: The influence of age, height, and body weight on cerebrospinal fluid amine metabolites and tryptophan in women. Biol Psychiatry 16:753–762, 1981

Banki CM, Bissette G, Arato M, et al: CSF corticotropin-releasing factor-like immunoreactivity in depression and schizophrenia. Am J Psychiatry 144:873–877, 1987

Berger PA, Faull KF, Kilkowski J, et al: CSF monoamine metabolites in depression and schizophrenia. Am J Psychiatry 137:174–180, 1980

Berrettini WH, Nurnberger JI, Scheinin M, et al: Cerebrospinal fluid and plasma monoamines and their metabolites in euthymic bipolar patients. Biol Psychiatry 20:257–269, 1985

Berrettini WH, Oxenstierna G, Sedvall G, et al: Characteristics of cerebrospinal fluid neuropeptides relevant to clinical research. Psychiatry Res 25:349–359, 1988

Carroll BJ, Feinberg M, Greden JF, et al: A specific laboratory test for the diagnosis of melancholia: standardization, validation, and clinical utility. Arch Gen Psychiatry 38:15–22, 1981

Endicott J, Spitzer R: A diagnostic interview: the Schedule for Affective Disorders and Schizophrenia. Arch Gen Psychiatry 35:837–844, 1979

Gerner RH, Fairbanks L, Anderson GM, et al: CSF neurochemistry in depressed, manic, and schizophrenic patients compared with that of normal controls. Am J Psychiatry 141:1533–1540, 1984

Gibbons RD, Davis JM: Consistent evidence for a biological subtype of depression characterized by low CSF monoamine levels. Acta Psychiatr Scand 74:8–12, 1986

Gjerris A, Werdelin L, Rafaelsen OJ, et al: CSF dopamine increased in depression: CSF dopamine, noradrenaline and their metabolites in depressed patients and in controls. J Affective Disord 13:279–286, 1987

Gold P, Loriaux D, Roy A, et al: Responses to corticotropin-releasing hormone in the hypercortisolism of depression and Cushing's disease. N Engl J Med 314:1329–1335, 1986

Koslow SH, Maas JW, Bowden CL, et al: CSF and urinary biogenic amines and metabolites in depression and mania. Arch Gen Psychiatry 40:999–1010, 1983

Nemeroff C, Widerlov E, Bisette G, et al: Elevated concentrations of CSF corticotropin-releasing factor-like immunoreactivity in depressed patients. Science 226:1342–1345, 1984

Roy A, Pickar D, Linnoila M, et al: Cerebrospinal fluid monoamine and monoamine metabolite concentrations in melancholia. Psychiatry Res 15:281–292, 1985

Sapolsky RM: Hypercortisolism among socially subordinate wild baboons originates at the CNS level. Arch Gen Psychiatry 46:1047–1051, 1989

Stahl SM: Can CSF measures distinguish among schizophrenia, depression, movement disorders, and dementia? Psychopharmacol Bull 21:396–399, 1985

Standish-Barry HMAS, Bouras N, Hale AS, et al: Ventricular size and CSF transmitter metabolite concentrations in severe endogenous depression. Br J Psychiatry 148:386–392, 1986

Stokes PE, Pick GR, Stoll PM, et al: Pituitary-adrenal function in depressed patients: resistance to dexamethasone suppression. J Psychiatr Res 12:271–282, 1975

Traskman-Bendz L, Asberg M, Bertilsson L, et al: CSF monoamine metabolites of depressed patients during illness and after recovery. Acta Psychiatr Scand 69:333–342, 1984

Widerlöv E, Bissette G, Nemiroff EB: Monoamine metabolites, corticotropin releasing factor and somatostatin as CSF markers in depressed patients. J Affective Disord 14:99–107, 1988

Chapter 5

Cellular Immune Changes in Stress and Depression: Role of Corticotropin-Releasing Factor and Endogenous Opioid Peptides

Michael Irwin, M.D.

D epressive states and distressing life experiences are associated with reduced cellular immune responses. In this chapter, I discuss the purported mechanisms by which the central nervous system might modulate immunity through activation of either the pituitary-adrenal axis or the autonomic nervous system. In addition, a model that involves the use of central corticotropin-releasing factor (CRF) is summarized in an effort to understand how the brain integrates biologic actions in response to stress and coordinates changes in immunity. An overview of the components of the cellular immune system is first provided. Then, in vitro correlates of immune activity used to measure the function of immune cells are described.

CELLULAR IMMUNITY

The function of an organism's immune system is to discriminate self cells from nonself cells, protecting the host from invasion by pathogens, such as viruses and bacteria, or from abnormal internal cells, such as cancer cells (Cohn 1985; Hood et al. 1985). The organs of the mammalian immune system include the thymus, spleen, and lymph nodes (Hood et al. 1985; Paul 1984). The working cells of the

This work was supported by a VA Merit Review grant, a Clinical Research on Alcoholism grant, NIMH Grant R29-MH44275-02, and UCSD Mental Health Research Center Grant MH30914. It was partly supported by NIMH Grants MH44275-01 and MH30914, the San Diego VA Clinical Research Center on Alcoholism, and a VA Merit Review. The work described in this chapter was done as part of my employment with the U.S. federal government and is in the public domain. Parts of this chapter have been previously published.

105

immune system are represented by three distinct populations—T cells, B cells, and natural killer (NK) cells (Hood et al. 1985; Paul 1984; Ritz 1989). Two important components of the cellular immune response are the cytotoxic T cell and the NK cell.

The cytotoxic T cell is characterized by its ability to seek out and destroy either cells infected with viruses or tumor cells that have acquired foreign nonself antigens (Henney and Gillis 1984; Zinkernagel and Doherty 1979). In the development of the cytotoxic T cell response, a foreign antigen is first incorporated onto the surface of an antigen-presenting cell, such as a macrophage. After the antigen is presented to the T cell and bound by a specific receptor on the T cell, then the T cell multiples and develops, becoming capable of attacking any cell that presents that specific foreign surface antigen. Other types of T lymphocytes, such as T helper cells, interact with the T killer cell to regulate its proliferative response to antigenic stimulation (Henney and Gillis 1984), mainly by the secretion of interleukin 2 (Gillis et al. 1981; Kern et al. 1981).

Distinct from the cytotoxic T cell, the NK cell is immunologically nonspecific and does not require sensitization to specific antigens (Lotzova and Herberman 1986; Trinchieri 1989). Thus, the NK cell responds to various cell surface markers, as long as the markers differ from self markers, and lyses a wide variety of cell types. Although the role of the NK cell in tumor surveillance remains controversial (Lotzova and Herberman 1986; Ritz 1989), substantial evidence demonstrates the importance of the NK cell in the control of herpes and cytomegalovirus infections in humans (Biron et al. 1989; Padgett et al. 1968; Sullivan et al. 1980) and animals (Bancroft et al. 1981; Bukowski et al. 1985; Habu et al. 1984).

Two immunologic assays that have been widely used to assess in vitro the function of the cell-mediated immune system are mitogen-induced lymphocyte proliferation and NK cell activity. Mitogen-induced lymphocyte stimulation evaluates the proliferative capacity of lymphocytes. Stimulation of lymphocytes in vitro with mitogens, such as the plant lectins concanavalin A or phytohemagglutinin (PHA), activates predominantly the T lymphocyte to divide. The proliferative response is quantitated by the cellular incorporation of radioactively labeled thymidine or idoxuridine into the newly synthesized DNA.

The other frequently used in vitro assessment of cellular immunity involves measurement of NK activity. Assay of NK lytic activity is carried out by the co-incubation of isolated lymphocytes with radioactively labeled tumor cells, and the release of radioactivity by the lysed target cells is proportionate to the activity of the effector NK cells (Herberman and Ortaldo 1981).

DEPRESSION, LIFE STRESS, AND ALTERED IMMUNITY

Clinically depressed patients and persons with depressive symptoms who are undergoing severe life stress appear to show a reduction in cellular immunity. In clinical studies of immune function in depression, the lymphocytes of depressed patients show a suppressed ability to respond to mitogenic stimulation (Darko et al. 1988; Kronfol et al. 1983; Schleifer et al. 1985) as well as a reduction of natural cytolytic activity compared with cells obtained from age-matched control subjects (Irwin and Gillin 1987; Irwin et al. 1987a, 1990a; Mohl et al. 1987; Nerozzi et al. 1989; Urich et al. 1988). Although not all studies have found depression-related alterations in immunity (Albrecht et al. 1985; Schleifer et al. 1989), it is possible that subgroups of depressed patients may be at greater risk to show changes in the immune system. In this regard, severity of depressive symptoms, age (Schleifer et al. 1989), and history of alcohol abuse (Irwin et al. 1990b) are all factors that are likely to contribute to the immune alterations found in depressed patients.

A similar suppression of cellular immune measures has been identified in persons who are anticipating or have experienced the death of a spouse (Bartrop et al. 1977; Irwin et al. 1987b, 1987c; Schleifer et al. 1983), in family care givers of patients with Alzheimer's disease (Kiecolt-Glaser et al. 1987), and in students undergoing academic examinations (Kiecolt-Glaser et al. 1984).

STRESS AND IMMUNE DYSFUNCTION: ANIMAL STUDIES

Behavioral responsiveness to inescapable aversive stimulation has provided an animal model to investigate clinical depression (Weiss et al. 1981). Aversive stressors—such as sound exposure (Irwin et al. 1989; Monjan and Collector 1977), rotation (Kandil and Borysenko 1987; Riley 1981), intermittent shock (Keller et al. 1981, 1983; Shavit et al. 1984), and forced immobilization (Irwin and Hauger 1988)—affect immune responses in a manner that depends on their dose- and time-response profiles. For example, using an audiogenic stressor repeated at daily intervals, Irwin et al. (1989) replicated the findings of Monjan and Collector (1977), who found that the initial stress-induced immune suppression is followed by an increase or enhancement of natural cytotoxicity. In regard to the effects of a dose of the stressor, Keller et al. (1981) demonstrated a relationship between the intensity of an acute stressor and the degree of suppression of T cell function. A progressive decrease of PHA-induced stimulation is found in animals who receive low-level apparatus tail shock or high-level electric tail shock, respectively, compared with home cage controls (Keller et al. 1981).

In addition to the effects of stressor characteristics, the psychological state of the animal in response to the stressor has also been related to the immunologic consequences of the stress. Laudenslager et al. (1983) found that rats exposed to inescapable and uncontrollable electric tail shock had reduced lymphocyte activity, whereas animals who received the same total amount of shock but were able to terminate it did not show altered immunity. Furthermore, Mormede et al. (1988) reported on the influence of stress predictability; a warning stimulus preceding inescapable foot shock completely reversed the shock-induced suppression of lymphocytes. Thus, consistent with the clinical data, psychological distress, as measured by behavioral responses in animals, not merely the stressor, is correlated with a reduction of cellular immunity. However, the mechanisms by which the brain affects immune function have not been fully explored. In the following sections, I describe how the autonomic and neuroendocrine pathways might influence immune function.

NEURAL INFLUENCES ON CELLULAR IMMUNITY: AUTONOMIC NERVOUS SYSTEM

The autonomic nervous system is one pathway for communication from the brain to cells of the immune system. Anatomic studies have revealed an extensive presence of autonomic fibers in primary and secondary lymphoid organs (Bulloch and Pomerantz 1984; D. Felten et al. 1981, 1984, 1985, 1987). Following a pattern of classic anatomical connection, preganglionic cell bodies are found in the intermediolateral cell column of the spinal cord, whereas the ganglion cells are found in the sympathetic chain or in collateral ganglia (D. Felten et al. 1987). Immunohistochemical studies have demonstrated that nervous fibers enter the lymphoid organs, such as the spleen, along with the vasculature and then branch into the parenchyma (D. Felten et al. 1985) and areas in which lymphocytes (primarily T cells) reside (Ackerman et al. 1987; D. Felten et al. 1985). These noradrenergic fibers are not only adjacent to T cells but, at the electron-microscopic level, end in synaptic contacts with lymphocytes in the spleen (S. Felten and Olschowka 1987). These observations establish an anatomical link between the brain and the immune system and raise the question of whether the role of norepinephrine is to serve as a neurotransmitter or a neuromodulator of immune function.

Consistent with the hypothesis that norepinephrine is involved as a neurotransmitter in immunomodulation, norepinephrine is released within the spleen. Von Euler (1946) found that splenic nerve stimulation yields a release of norepinephrine. Furthermore, in vivo dialysis techniques document a 1-μM concentration of norepinephrine in the rat spleen (S. Felten et al. 1986), a concentration that is more than 100-fold higher than that found in blood, suggesting local release of norepinephrine within the spleen.

Lymphocytes are capable of receiving signals from the sympathetic neurons innervating lymphoid tissue. Adrenoreceptors that bind norepinephrine, epinephrine, and dopamine have been demonstrated on lymphocytes (Aaron and Molinoff 1982; Bidart et al. 1983; Brodde et al. 1981; Miles et al. 1981; Motulsky and Insel 1982; Williams et al. 1976). These β-receptors are linked to adenylate cyclase (Katz et al. 1982; Strom et al. 1977; Watson 1975) and appear to have a functional role in the modulation of cellular immunity. In vitro incubation of lymphocytes with varying concentrations of norepinephrine or epinephrine can decrease NK activity (Hellstrand et al. 1985) and mitogenic responses (Hadden et al. 1970). Because preincubation with a β-antagonist reverses the inhibitory effects of norepinephrine in vitro (Hellstrand et al. 1985), it is believed that β-adrenoreceptor binding mediates an inhibition of cellular immunity (Livnat et al. 1985). The potential role of the sympathetic nervous system in mediating immune processes in vivo is discussed later in this chapter.

PITUITARY-ADRENAL AXIS AND CELLULAR IMMUNITY

The neuroendocrine system might also exert influence on immune responses. The secretion of corticosteroids has long been considered to be the mechanism of stress-induced and/or depression-related suppression of immune function (Cupps and Fauci 1982; Munck et al. 1984; Parrillo and Fauci 1978; Riley 1981; Selye 1976). Specific intracytoplasmic corticosteroid receptors have been identified in normal human lymphocytes (Lippman and Barr 1977); they bind corticosteroids and appear to play a role in the regulation of cellular function through modulation of cyclic AMP levels (Parker et al. 1973). In vitro studies have further demonstrated that glucocorticoids can act to inhibit production of interleukin 2 in vitro, with a resulting suppression of lymphocyte responses to mitogenic stimulation (Gillis et al. 1979) and NK cell activity (antibody-dependent cytotoxicity is relatively refractory to glucocorticoids; Parrillo and Fauci 1978).

Despite pharmacological in vitro and in vivo studies that show a suppressive effect of corticosteroids on cell-mediated immune function, recent evidence in animals suggests that stress-induced increases in adrenocortical activity might not solely mediate changes in immune function. Acute administration of forced immobilization (Irwin and Hauger 1988) or audiogenic stress (Irwin et al. 1989) is capable of producing activation of adrenal steroid secretion, but neither acute stressor alters immune function as measured by NK cell activity. Furthermore, with repeated exposure to the stressor, pituitary adrenal activation is dissociated from a reduction in cytotoxicity (Irwin and Hauger 1988; Irwin et al. 1989). In addition, Keller et al. (1983, 1988) found that stress-induced suppression of lymphocyte function after unpredictable, unavoidable tail shock can occur in adrenalectomized and hypophysectomized animals.

Keller et al. (1983) determined whether the adrenal is required for stress-induced changes in immunity. As compared to responses in home cage controls, lymphocyte responses to PHA were significantly lower after tail shock in non-operated animals, in sham-adrenalectomized animals, and in adrenalectomized animals with steroid replacement. Stress-induced lymphopenia was prevented by adrenalectomy, but the secretion of corticosteroids was not required for stress-related suppression of lymphocyte responses to mitogens. Similarly, in a second study (Keller et al. 1988), hypophysectomy did not alter the effects of tail-shock stress to suppress peripheral blood PHA responses, although stress-induced lymphopenia and suppression of splenic NK activity appeared to be pituitary dependent.

Consistent with these animal studies that have suggested that neither alterations in lymphocyte responses to mitogenic stimulation nor a reduction of NK activity after stress is mediated by increased secretion of adrenal corticosteroids, clinical research has found a dissociation between adrenocortical activity and immunity in depressed patients and in stressed persons. In depressed patients, decreased lymphocyte responses to mitogens are not associated with dexamethasone nonsuppression (Kronfol and House 1985) or with increased excretion rate of urinary free cortisol (Kronfol et al. 1986). Furthermore, in bereavement, in which a reduction of NK activity has been demonstrated, these immunologic changes occur even in subjects who have plasma cortisol levels comparable to those of control subjects (Irwin et al. 1988a).

OPIOID PEPTIDES AND IMMUNOMODULATION

Opioid peptides have been increasingly implicated in immune regulation. Opioids secreted from peripheral sites, such as the pituitary or adrenal glands, can bind to opioid receptors on lymphocytes (Sibinga and Goldstein 1988) and potentially alter immune function in vivo

(Morley et al. 1987). In addition, evidence exists that opioids can act within the central nervous system to coordinate changes in immunity (Shavit et al. 1985).

Pharmacological evidence has shown that some cells of the immune system have opioid receptors, although the data remain tentative and fragmentary and few studies have reported on the saturability or stereospecificity of these binding sites (Sibinga and Goldstein 1988). One of the earliest reports that suggested opioid binding on immune cells was that of Wybran et al. (1979). Active rosetting of human T lymphocytes was affected by nanomolar concentrations of opioids. Morphine inhibited rosetting, whereas met-enkephalin stimulated it and both effects were blocked by naloxone. Other studies have expanded on these findings and have demonstrated, via radiolabeling techniques, specific opioid binding on human phagocytic leukocytes (Falke et al. 1985; Farrar 1984; Lopker et al. 1980), platelets (Mehrishi and Mills 1983), and lymphocytes (Ausiello and Roda 1984; Mehrishi and Mills 1983).

In vitro studies have shown that endogenous opioid peptides are able to influence the function of most cell types of the immune system. Whereas some of these effects are mediated by classical opiate receptor binding (i.e., they are naloxone reversible), other immunomodulating actions of β-endorphin are mediated through nonclassical opiate receptor binding (i.e., when β-endorphin is not bound through its amino terminus).

Two measures of cellular immunity, lymphocyte proliferation and NK activity, are affected in vitro by opioids. Johnson et al. (1982) found that α-endorphin, met-enkephalin, and leu-enkephalin (all with approximately equal potency) decreased the proliferation and antibody production of splenocytes in the plaque-forming assay, an effect that was blocked by naloxone. Confirming these results, Heijnen et al. (1986) demonstrated that (des-tyr) β-endorphin was also active in suppressing the plaque-forming cell response. Proliferation induced by PHA is affected by opioid peptides, although stimulatory (Bocchini et al. 1983; Farrar 1984; Gilman et al. 1982; Gilmore and Weiner 1989) and inhibitory (McCain et al. 1986; Puppo et al. 1985) effects have been reported. The β-endorphin enhancement of mitogen-induced lymphocyte proliferation and of interleukin 2 production was not blocked by the specific opiate antagonist naloxone (Gilmore and Weiner 1988).

In regard to natural cytotoxic activity, several studies have reported an enhancing effect of lytic activity by opioids in vitro. By using a standard chromium lysis method with K562 tumor cells as targets, Mathews et al. (1983) reported a naloxone-reversible enhancement of human natural cytotoxicity. Enhancement of NK activity occurred at very low concentrations of β-endorphin (10 fM) and of met-enkephalin (10 pM). Although Kay et al. (1984) also found a similar enhancement of NK function, β-endorphin had an inverted U-shaped dose response and was effective only between 1 and 100 nM. Similar results were described by Mandler et al. (1986), who used 10–100 pM β-endorphin and blocked the enhancement by naloxone. Finally, Oleson and Johnson (1988) described a bidirectional effect of the enkephalins and selective opiate agonists on human NK activity. In subjects with low (below the median) NK activity, enkephalin at 10^{-10} M stimulated cytotoxic activity, whereas the cytolytic activity of cells from the high group were inhibited by similar doses of enkephalin (Oleson and Johnson 1988). Recent evidence suggests that endorphins stimulate NK activity through the (6–9) amino acid region, the α-helix portion of β-endorphin (Kay et al. 1987).

Although the physiological importance of opioid modulation of immune function cannot be adduced with confidence, systemic administration of opioids and the release of opiate peptides after stress appear to be related to changes of NK cytotoxicity in animals. Consistent with the enhancing effect of endorphin in vitro, Irwin and Hauger (1988) reported a positive correlation between secretion of β-endorphin and increases in splenic NK activity after acute administration of forced immobilization in rats. In comparison with these data, however, opposite effects of opiates on NK activity were found in rats repeatedly administered intermittent inescapable foot shock for four consecutive days (Shavit et al. 1984). This intermittent shock paradigm resulted in a significant suppression of NK activity, which was antagonized by the preadministration of naltrexone. In addition, daily injection of morphine for four days at doses of 10, 30, or 50 mg/kg also produced a similar suppression of cytotoxicity (Shavit et al. 1984, 1985, 1986). These data suggest that repeated release of opiates induces a suppression of cytotoxicity in vivo.

Central mechanisms may mediate, at least in part, the effects of systemic administration of morphine to suppress NK activity. In addition to direct peripheral effects, systemic morphine might cross the blood-brain barrier to act within the brain, activating the pituitary adrenal axis (Rivier et al. 1977) or the autonomic nervous system (Van Loon and Appel 1981). To examine the role of the central nervous system in opiate-induced modulation of NK cytotoxicity, Shavit et al. (1986) gave small doses of morphine centrally. These studies show that the effective dose of morphine given into the cerebral ventricle is a thousand times smaller than that required when given systemically. Moreover, a morphine analogue that does not cross the blood-brain barrier to enter the central nervous system was not effective in altering NK activity. Finally, intracerebral infusion of morphine into the periaqueductal gray, but not other brain regions, produced a suppression of NK activity (Weber and Pert 1989). These data suggest that acute doses of opiates can alter cytotoxicity through a central action site.

Although the evidence remains circumstantial and contradictory, opiates also correlate with immune changes in humans. For example, chronic opiate exposure was associated with a depressed frequency of T cells and with reduced in vitro responsiveness of T cells to mitogenic stimulation in street heroin addicts and in a population maintained on methadone (McDonough et al. 1980). In contrast, the in vivo administration of enkephalins might have immunoenhancing effects. Preliminary in vivo studies of healthy human volunteers and several acquired immune deficiency syndrome patients suggest an enhancement of T cell proliferation and NK activity (Plotnikoff et al. 1986a, 1986b; Wybran et al. 1987). Oleson et al. (1989) further examined the ability of leu-enkephalin to modify NK activity in subjects with and without human immunodeficiency virus (HIV) infection. The cytotoxicity of NK cells was consistently enhanced in seven subjects with HIV infection, whereas subjects without HIV infection ($n = 4$) demonstrated a suppression or no change in NK activity. However, the effects of enkephalins on cellular immunity may be transient and not clinically efficacious. In an evaluation of immunomodulating effects of met-enkephalin (10 μg/kg) given three times weekly for up to 12 weeks, increases in interleukin 2 production were seen 30 minutes and 24 hours after infusion in some patients, but no differences were found between pre- and post-treatment values (Zunich and Kirkpatrick 1988). Furthermore, there were no significant changes in numbers of circulating T cells of any phenotype or in T cell responses to mitogens or antigens (Zunich and Kirkpatrick 1988).

In summary, opioid peptides act on receptors of cells of the immune system and are capable of modulating aspects of cellular immunity, particularly NK activity. In addition, the immune system may be modulated in vivo by the action of endogenous opioid peptides within the central nervous system.

CENTRAL MODULATION OF IMMUNE FUNCTION: ROLE OF CRF

It is tempting to speculate that central changes in CRF might coordinate a reduction of immunity in depression and severe life stress. In support of such speculation, increased concentrations of CRF have been found in the cerebrospinal fluid of depressed patients (Nemeroff et al. 1984), and CRF has been postulated as a physiological central nervous system regulator that integrates biological responses to stress (Axelrod and Reisine 1984; Taylor and Fishman 1988). Thus, CRF is expected to alter not only endocrine function (Vale et al. 1981) but also autonomic (Brown et al. 1982) and visceral functions (Lenz et al. 1987), including immune function (Irwin et al. 1987d) (Figure 5-1).

Although neuroanatomic studies of the brain have shown that the greatest density of CRF immunoreactive cells and fibers are found in the paraventricular nucleus of the hypothalamus, immunohistochemical studies have revealed a wide distribution of CRF throughout the brain (Olschowka et al. 1982a, 1982b; Swanson et al. 1983). Furthermore, CRF receptors that are relatively absent in the hypothalamus have been autoradiographically mapped to numerous other

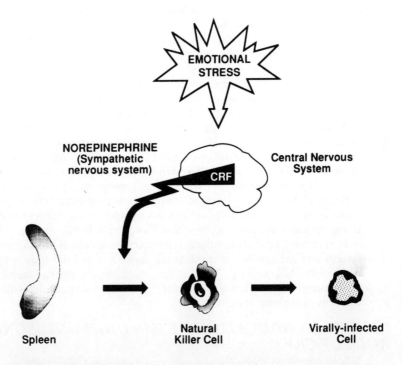

Figure 5-1. Hypothetical model that illustrates release of corticotropin-releasing factor (CRF) in brain following stress to activate the autonomic nervous system and reduce natural killer cytotoxicity.

extrahypothalamic structures that are related to the limbic system and control the autonomic nervous system (De Souza et al. 1984; Wynn et al. 1984). Thus, in addition to its well-established role as a hypothalamic regulator of the pituitary secretion of ACTH and β-endorphin (Vale et al. 1981), CRF may also act directly in the central nervous system at extrahypothalamic sites. Correspondingly, studies have shown that exogenous CRF administered to animals induces numerous changes in brain function. Intraventricular CRF increases the firing rate of the locus coeruleus (Valentino et al. 1983), activates the autonomic nervous system as reflected by increased plasma concentrations of norepinephrine and epinephrine (Fisher et al. 1982), and produces a pattern of behavioral responses, such as decreased feeding and increased locomotor activity (Britton et al. 1982; Sherman and Kalin 1985; Sutton et al. 1982).

Based on interest in understanding the central processes involved in the pathogenesis of immune impairment that is associated with depression, the role of intraventricular CRF in the regulation of immune function in the rat has been examined. The data of Irwin et al. (1987d) demonstrate that central administration of CRF produces a dose-dependent suppression of NK activity that appears specific and independent of direct systemic mechanisms.

Dose-Response Profile of Intraventricular CRF

The effect of intraventricular CRF on rat splenic NK activity has been examined with doses of CRF that produce behavioral, pituitary, and autonomoic actions similar to the responses found in animals subjected to some types of stressors (Irwin et al. 1987d). Measurement of NK activity was carried out one hour after intraventricular infusion, a time interval found to result in maximal increases in locomotor activity, plasma norepinephrine, and corticosterone levels. In the first study involving the administration of intraventricular CRF, a dose-dependent reduction of NK activity was found across three CRF doses—.1, .5, and 1.0 µg. The highest dose of intraventricular CRF (1.0 µg) significantly ($P<.05$) decreased splenic NK activity to 74+3.1% of the saline-treated group. This finding demonstrated that CRF is capable of modulating immune function in vivo, but it did not address whether the action of intraventricular CRF was caused by a central action of the neuropeptide or a consequence of CRF being distributed from the brain into the peripheral circulation to act directly on lymphocytes.

Lack of Direct Systemic Action of CRF

Additional experiments have tested the possibility that CRF might have a direct peripheral action on NK cells, which contributes to the immunosuppressive effect of centrally administered doses. In these experiments, CRF was administered subcutaneously in three doses— 5.0, 10.0, and 20.0 µg/kg. It is difficult to equate the dose administered peripherally with that given centrally, but the lowest systemic dose of 5.0 µg/kg is roughly equivalent per rat to the 1.0 µg intracerebroventricular (ICV) CRF dose, and the 20 µg/kg systemic CRF dose represents about 6.0 µg per rat. Thus, if central CRF (1.0 µg ICV) is crossing the blood-brain barrier to act peripherally on the NK cell, then 5.0 µg/kg CRF administered systemically should have a similar effect; however, the 5.0 µg/kg dose of CRF administered subcutaneously had no significant effect on NK cell activity.

Although there is a trend for NK activity to be reduced after administration of the 20.0 µg/kg dose, this decrease is not statistically significant. At such a high systemic dose, it is possible that CRF crosses the blood-brain barrier from the peripheral circulation and enters the brain. Thus, subcutaneous CRF, even in high doses, does not appear to alter NK activity significantly.

To examine further the potential effect of CRF on lymphocytes, an additional study was carried out in which rat splenic lymphocytes were incubated for one hour in vitro with CRF at a range of concentrations from 10^{-6} M to 10^{-12} M. Throughout the range of CRF concentrations, NK activity was similar to the values found in untreated cells, a result demonstrated in three separate experiments. The lack of effect of CRF on NK cells is supported by the lack of CRF binding on purified lymphocyte preparations, even though CRF receptors have been identified on monocytes (Webster and de Souza 1988; Webster et al. 1990).

These findings indicate that the direct application of CRF does not acutely reduce NK activity and that CRF is unlikely to cross the blood-brain barrier in sufficient doses to alter cytotoxicity. Both of these findings support the hypothesis that the immunosuppressive effect of CRF is centrally mediated and independent of direct systemic mechanisms.

Central Specificity of CRF Action

The immunosuppressive effect of centrally administered exogenous CRF may result from the nonspecific effects of the neuropeptide. To address the specificity of this action of CRF, the CRF antagonist α-helical (9-41) was coadministered with CRF. The CRF antagonist was administered alone or in combination with intraventricular CRF. In another group of rats, the antagonist was injected peripherally, followed by a central dose of CRF. Rats coadministered intra-ventricular CRF and the CRF antagonist showed values of NK activity comparable to those observed in saline-treated rats. Thus, central administration of the CRF antagonist significantly attenuated the action of central CRF. In contrast, when a systemic dose of the antagonist (.5 mg/kg body weight) was coadministered with in-traventricular CRF (1.0 µg), values of NK activity were significantly lower ($P<.05$) than those in saline-treated controls; systemic administration of the CRF antagonist failed to alter the suppression of NK activity induced by central CRF.

Corticotropin-Releasing Factor Reduction of NK Activity: Role of Autonomic Nervous System

Central administration of CRF produces an acute decrease in splenic NK activity and provides a model to study the relationship between central processes and immune cells via efferent outflow pathways of the neuroendocrine and autonomic nervous systems. The role of the autonomic nervous system in mediating CRF-induced suppression of NK cytotoxicity was explored first (Irwin et al. 1988b), because central CRF produces an activation of sympathetic outflow, the spleen is extensively innervated by sympathetic fibers, and norepinephrine inhibits NK activity (S. Felten et al. 1988). By using the peripheral ganglionic blocker chlorisondamine, the impact of autonomic activation in directly mediating CRF-induced suppression of NK activity has been examined. Chlorisondamine administered to animals that receive intraventricular CRF significantly antagonized ($P<.05$) CRF-induced elevations of plasma concentrations of norepinephrine and epinephrine and completely abolished the immunosuppressive effect of CRF on NK activity. Although chlorisondamine given alone produced a modest increase in cytotoxicity compared with the saline controls, this intrinsic effect of chlorisondamine was not statistically significant. These bindings suggest that ganglionic blockade is cap-able of antagonizing the action of central CRF and that autonomic activation is one pathway that communicates the action of CRF in the brain to the immune system.

Neuroendocrine Outflow and CRF Action

The other major efferent through which CRF might act to suppress NK activity is the pituitary-adrenal axis. To separate the influence of the sympathetic activation from that involving the pituitary-adrenal axis, an additional study was carried out; it involved the concurrent measurement of NK activity and the neuroendocrine variables in CRF-treated rats with and without chlorisondamine pretreatment

(Irwin et al. 1988b). Again, although chlorisondamine significantly antagonized CRF suppression of NK activity, it did not significantly attenuate CRF-induced elevations of ACTH and corticosterone. Levels of ACTH and corticosterone in rats treated with CRF and chlorisondamine were comparable to those found in rats treated only with CRF. Both CRF treatment groups (with and without ganglionic blockade) demonstrate a significant activation of the pituitary-adrenal axis, but only the treatment with CRF alone suppressed NK activity. Thus, ganglionic blockade is capable of antagonizing the reduction of cytotoxicity, but that effect is dissociated from the activation of the pituitary-adrenal axis. Additional experiments have suggested that the increased secretion of glucocorticoids does not significantly contribute to CRF suppression of NK cytotoxicity. Intraventricular CRF administered to animals, in whom synthesis of corticosterone is blocked pharmacologically by preadministering metyrapone and aminoglutethimide before CRF infusion, produces a reduction of NK activity comparable to that in animals that have not undergone similar blockade of glucocorticoid synthesis.

These data, evaluating the role of the autonomic nervous system and neuroendocrine systems in mediating the effects of CRF, demonstrate that the autonomic nervous system is a salient efferent pathway by which CRF suppresses NK activity; blockade of this outflow completely antagonizes the action of CRF. Moreover, CRF immunosuppression appears independent of the activation of the pituitary gland. Significant increases of plasma levels of these hormones can occur without necessarily reducing NK activity.

SUMMARY

In this chapter, I have demonstrated several points. Clinical studies have clarified that a reduction of immune function is associated with psychological processes in persons undergoing severe, adverse life events; reduced NK activity is correlated with the severity of depressive symptoms in both stressed persons and depressed patients. Preclinical studies have demonstrated an extensive autonomic nervous innervation of lymphoid tissue. Furthermore, a series of studies has also shown that the neuroendocrine system and opiate peptides can influence cellular immunity. In an attempt to understand the link between the central nervous system and immune function, clinical research has been extended to an animal model that involves the central administration of CRF. Intraventricular CRF has been found to reduce NK activity in addition to its abilities to coordinate a pattern of behavioral, pituitary, and autonomic responses similar to those found in animals exposed to some types of stressors. The central action of CRF and the finding that ganglionic blockade completely antagonizes the suppression of NK activity induced by CRF provide direct evidence that changes in the brain are communicated to NK cells via the autonomic nervous system.

REFERENCES

Aaron RD, Molinoff PB: Changes in the density of beta adrenergic receptors in rat lymphocytes, heart, and lung after chronic treatment with propranolol. J Pharm Exp Ther 221:439–443, 1982

Ackerman KD, Felten SY, Bellinger DL, et al: Noradrenergic sympathetic innervation of spleen and lymph nodes in relation to specific cellular compartments. Prog Immunol 6:588–600, 1987

Albrecht J, Helderman J, Schlesser M, et al: A controlled study of cellular immune function in affective disorders before and during somatic therapy. Psychiatry Res 15:185–193, 1985

Ausiello CM, Roda LG: Leuenkephalin binding to cultured human T lymphocytes. Cell Biol Int Rep 8:353–362, 1984

Axelrod J, Reisine TD: Stress hormones: their interaction and regulation. Science 224:452–459, 1984

Bancroft GJ, Shellam GR, Chalmer JE: Genetic influences on the augmentation of natural killer cells (NK) during murine cytomegalovirus infection: correlation with patterns of resistance. J Immunol 124:988–994, 1981

Bartrop RW, Lazarus L, Luckherst E, et al: Depressed lymphocyte function after bereavement. Lancet 1:834–836, 1977

Bidart JM, Motte PH, Assicot M, et al: Catechol-O-methyltransferase activity and aminergic binding sites distribution in human peripheral blood lymphocyte subpopulations. Clin Immunol Immunopathol 26:1–9, 1983

Biron CA, Byron KS, Sullivan JL: Severe herpes virus infections in an adolescent without natural killer cells. N Engl J Med 320:1732–1735, 1989

Bocchini G, Bonanno G, Canivari A: Influence of morphine and naloxone on human peripheral blood T-lymphocytes. Drug Alcohol Depend 11:233–237, 1983

Britton KT, Koob GF, Rivier J: ICV-CRF enhanced behavioral effects of novelty. Life Sci 31:363–367, 1982

Brodde OE, Engel G, Hoyer D, et al: The beta-adrenergic receptor in human lymphocytes: subclassification by the use of a new radio-ligand (+)–[125]iodocyanopindolol. Life Sci 29:2189–2198, 1981

Brown MR, Fisher LA, Spiess J, et al: Corticotropin-releasing factor: actions on the sympathetic nervous system and metabolism. Endocrinology 111:928–931, 1982

Bukowski JF, Warner JF, Dennert G, et al: Adoptive transfer studies demonstrating the antiviral affect of natural killer cells in vivo. J Exp Med 131:1531–1538, 1985

Bulloch K, Pomerantz W: Autonomic nervous system innervation of thymic-related lymphoid tissue in wild-type and nude mice. J Comp Neurol 228:57–68, 1984

Cohn M: What are the "must" elements of immune responsiveness? in Neural Modulation of Immunity. Edited by Guillemin R, Cohn M, Melnechuk T. New York, Raven, 1985, pp 3–25

Cupps TR, Fauci AS: Corticosteroid-mediated immunoregulation in man. Immunological Rev 65:133–155, 1982

Darko DF, Gillin JC, Bulloch SC, et al: Immune cells and the hypothalamic-pituitary axis in major depression. Psychiatry Res 25:173–179, 1988

De Souza EB, Perrin MH, Insel TR, et al: CRF receptors in rat forebrain: autoradiographic identification. Science 224:1449–1451, 1984

Falke NE, Fischer EG, Martin R: Stereospecific opiate binding in living human polymorphonuclear leucocytes. Cell Biol Int Rep 9:1041–1047, 1985

Farrar WL: Endorphin modulation of lymphokine activity. Dev Neurosci 18:159–165, 1984

Felten DL, Overhage JM, Felten SY, et al: Noradrenergic sympathetic innervation of lymphoid tissue systems. Brain Res Bull 7:595–612, 1981

Felten DL, Livnat S, Felten SY, et al: Sympathetic innervation of lymph nodes in mice. Brain Res Bull 13:693–699, 1984

Felten DL, Felten SY, Carlson SL, et al: Noradrenergic and peptidergic innervation of lymphoid tissue. J Immunol 135:765s–775s, 1985

Felten DL, Felten SY, Bellinger DL, et al: Noradrenergic sympathetic neural interactions with the immune system: structure and function. Immunological Rev 100:225–260, 1987

Felten SY, Olschowka J: Noradrenergic sympathetic innervation of the spleen, II: tyrosine hydroxylase (TH)-positive nerve terminals form synaptic-like contacts on lymphocytes in the splenic white pulp. J Neurosci Res 18:37–48, 1987

Felten SY, Housel J, Felten DL: Use of in vivo dialysis for evaluation of splenic norepinephrine and serotonin. Soc Neurosci Abstr 12:1065, 1986

Felten SY, Felten DC, Bellinger DC, et al: Noradrenergic sympathetic innervation of lymphoid organs. Prog Allergy 43:14–36, 1988

Fisher LA, Rivier J, Rivier C, et al: CRF: central effects on mean arterial pressure and heart rate in rats. Endocrinology 11:2222–2224, 1982

Gillis S, Crabtree GR, Smith KA: Glucocorticoid-induced inhibition of T cell growth factor production, I: the effect on mitogen-induced lymphocyte proliferation. J Immunol 123:1624–1631, 1979

Gillis S, Gillis AE, Henney CS: Monoclonal antibody directed against interleukin-2, I: inhibition of T-lymphocyte mitogenesis, and the in vitro differentiation of alloreactive cytolytic T-cells. J Exp Med 154:983–987, 1981

Gilman SC, Schwartz JM, Milner RJ, et al: B-endorphin enhances lymphocyte proliferative responses. Proc Natl Acad Sci USA 79:4226–4230, 1982

Gilmore W, Weiner LP: B-endorphin enhances interleukin-2 (IL-2) production in murine lymphocytes. J Neuroimmunol 18:125–138, 1988

Gilmore W, Weiner LP: The opioid specificity of beta-endorphin enhancement of murine lymphocyte proliferation. Immunopharmacology 17:19–30, 1989

Habu S, Akamatsu K, Tamaoki N, et al: In vivo significance of NK cells on resistance against virus (HSV-1) infections in mice. J Immunol 133:2743–2747, 1984

Hadden JW, Hadden EM, Middleton E: Lymphocyte host transformation, I: demonstration of adrenergic receptors in human peripheral lymphocytes. J Cell Immunol 1:583–595, 1970

Heijnen CJ, Bevers C, Kavelaars A, et al: Effect of α-endorphin on the antigen-induced primary antibody response of human blood B cells in vitro. J Immunol 136:213–216, 1986

Hellstrand K, Hermodsson S, Strannegard O: Evidence for a beta adrenoceptor mediated regulation of human natural killer cells. J Immunol 134:4095–4099, 1985

Henney CS, Gillis S: Cell-mediated cytotoxicity, in Fundamental Immunology. Edited by Paul WE. New York, Raven, 1984, pp 669–684

Herberman RB, Ortaldo JR: Natural killer cells: their role in defenses against disease. Science 214:24–30, 1981

Hood LE, Weisman IL, Wood HB, et al: Immunology. Menlo Park, CA, Benjamin Cummings, 1985

Irwin MR, Gillin JC: Impaired natural killer cell activity among depressed patients. Psychiatry Res 20:181–182, 1987

Irwin MR, Hauger RL: Adaptation to chronic stress: temporal pattern of immune and neuroendocrine correlates. Neuropsychopharmacology 1:239–243, 1988

Irwin M, Smith TL, Gillin JC: Reduced natural killer cytotoxicity in depressed patients. Life Sci 41:2127–2133, 1987a

Irwin M, Daniels M, Bloom E, et al: Life events, depressive symptoms and immune function. Am J Psychiatry 44:437–441, 1987b

Irwin MR, Daniels M, Smith TL, et al: Impaired natural killer cell activity during bereavement. Brain Behav Immun 1:98–104, 1987c

Irwin MR, Britton KT, Vale W: Central corticotropin releasing factor suppresses natural killer cell activity. Brain Behav Immun 1:81–87, 1987d

Irwin M, Daniels M, Risch SC, et al: Plasma cortisol and natural killer cell activity during bereavement. Biol Psychiatry 24:173–178, 1988a

Irwin MR, Hauger RL, Brown MR, et al: Corticotropin-releasing factor activates the autonomic nervous system and reduces natural cytotoxicity. Am J Physiol Integ Reg Mechanisms 255:R744–747, 1988b

Irwin MR, Segal D, Hauger RL, et al: Individual behavioral and neuroendocrine differences in responsiveness to repeated audiogenic stress. Pharmacol Biochem Behav 32:913–917, 1989

Irwin MR, Patterson T, Smith TL, et al: Reduction of immune function in life stress and depression. Biol Psychiatry 27:22–30, 1990a

Irwin MR, Caldwell C, Smith TL, et al: Major depressive disorder, alcoholism, and reduced natural killer cell cytotoxicity: role of severity of depressive symptoms and alcohol consumption. Arch Gen Psychiatry 47:713–719, 1990b

Johnson HM, Smith EM, Torres BA, et al: Regulation of the in vitro antibody response by neuroendocrine hormones. Proc Natl Acad Sci USA 79:4171–4174, 1982

Kandil O, Borysenko M: Decline of natural killer cell target binding and lytic activity in mice exposed to rotation stress. Health Psychol 6:89–99, 1987

Katz P, Zaytoun AM, Fauci AS: Mechanisms of human cell-mediated cytotoxicity, I: modulation of natural killer cell activity by cyclic nucleotides. J Immunol 129:287–296, 1982

Kay N, Allen J, Morley JE: Endorphins stimulate normal human peripheral blood lymphocyte natural killer activity. Life Sci 35:53–59, 1984

Kay N, Morley JE, Van Ree JM: Enhancement of human lymphocyte natural killing function by non-opioid fragments of beta-endorphin. Life Sci 40:1083–1087, 1987

Keller S, Weiss JM, Schleifer SJ, et al: Suppression of immunity by stress: effects of a graded series of stressors on lymphocytes stimulation in the rat. Science 213:1397–1400, 1981

Keller S, Weiss JM, Schleifer SJ, et al: Stress induced suppression of immunity in adrenalectomized rats. Science 221:1301–1304, 1983

Keller SE, Schleifer SJ, Liotta AS, et al: Stress-induced alterations of immunity in hypophysectomized rats. Proc Natl Acad Sci USA 85:9297–9301, 1988

Kern DE, Gillis S, Okada M, et al: The role of interleukin-2 (IL-2) in the differentiation of cytotoxic T cells: the effect of monoclonal anti-IL-2 antibody and absorption with IL-2 dependent T cell lines. J Immunol 127:1323–1328, 1981

Kiecolt-Glaser JK, Garner W, Speicher C, et al: Psychosocial modifiers of immunocompetence in medical students. Psychosom Med 46:7–14, 1984

Kiecolt-Glaser JK, Glaser R, Shuttleworth EC, et al: Chronic stress and immunity in family caregivers of Alzheimer's disease victims. Psychosom Med 49:523–535, 1987

Kronfol Z, House JD: Depression, hypothalamic-pituitary adrenocortical activity and lymphocyte function. Psychopharmacol Bull 21:476–478, 1985

Kronfol Z, Silva J, Greden J: Impaired lymphocyte function in depressive illness. Life Sci 33:241–247, 1983

Kronfol Z, Hover JD, Silva J, et al: Depression, urinary free cortisol excretion, and lymphocyte function. Br J Psychiatry 148:70–73, 1986

Laudenslager ML, Ryan SM, Drugan RC, et al: Coping and immunosuppression: inescapable but not escapable shock suppresses lymphocyte proliferation. Science 221:568–570, 1983

Lenz HJ, Raedler A, Greten H, et al: CRF initiates biological action within the brain that are observed in response to stress. Am J Physiol 252:34–39, 1987

Lippman M, Barr R: Glucocorticoid receptors in purified subpopulations of human peripheral blood lymphocytes. J Immunol 118:1977–1981, 1977

Livnat S, Felten SJ, Carlton SL, et al: Involvement of peripheral and central catecholamine systems in neural-immune interactions. Neuroimmunology 10:5–30, 1985

Lopker A, Abood LG, Hoss W, et al: Stereoselective muscarinic acetylcholine and opiate receptors in human phagocytic leukocytes. Biochem Pharmacol 29:1361–1365, 1980

Lotzova E, Herberman RB: Immunobiology of NK Cells II. Boca Raton, FL, CRC Press, 1986

Mandler RN, Biddison WE, Mandler R, et al: β-endorphin augments the cytolytic activity and interferon production of natural killer cells. J Immunol 136:934–939, 1986

Mathews PM, Froelich CJ, Sibbitt WL, et al: Enhancement of natural cytotoxicity by β-endorphin. J Immunol 130:1658–1662, 1983

McCain HW, Lamster IB, Bilotta J: Modulation of human T-cell suppressor activity by beta endorphin and glycyl-L-glutamine. Int J Immunopharmacol 8:443–446, 1986

McDonough RJ, Madden JJ, Falek A, et al: Alteration of T and null lymphocyte frequencies in the peripheral blood of human opiate addicts: in vivo evidence for opiate receptor sites on T lymphocytes. J Immunol 125:2539–2543, 1980

Mehrishi JN, Mills IH: Opiate receptors on lymphocytes and platelets in man. Clin Immunol Immunopathol 27:240–249, 1983

Miles K, Quintans E, Chelmicka-Schorr E: The sympathetic nervous system modulates antibody responses to thymus-independent antigens. J Neuroimmunol 1:101–105, 1981

Mohl PC, Huang L, Bowden C, et al: Natural killer cell activity in major depression (letter). Am J Psychiatry 144:1619, 1987

Monjan AA, Collector MI: Stress-induced modulation of the immune response. Science 196:307–308,1977

Morley JE, Kay NE, Solomon GF, et al: Minireview: neuropeptides: conductors of the immune orchestra. Life Sci 41:527–544, 1987

Mormede P, Dantzer R, Michaud B, et al: Influence of stressor predictability and behavioral control on lymphocyte reactivity, antibody responses and neuroendocrine activation in rats. Physiol Behav 43:577–583, 1988

Motulsky HJ, Insel PA: Medical progress: adrenergic receptors in man: direct identification, physiologic regulation, and clinical alterations. N Engl J Med 307:18–29, 1982

Munck A, Guyre PM, Holbrook NJ: Physiological functions of glucocorticoids in stress and their relation to pharmacologic actions. Endocr Rev 5:25–44, 1984

Nemeroff CB, Widerlov E, Bissette G, et al: Elevated concentrations of CSF corticotropin-releasing-factor-like immunoreactivity in depressed patients. Science 226:1342–1344, 1984

Nerozzi D, Santoni A, Bersani G, et al: Reduced natural killer cell activity in major depression: neuroendocrine implications. Psychoneuroendocrinology 14:295–302, 1989

Oleson DR, Johnson DR: Regulation of human natural cytotoxicity by enkephalins and selective opiate agonists. Brain Behav Immun 2:171–186, 1988

Oleson D, Grierson H, Goldsmith J, et al: Augmentation of natural cytotoxicity by leucine enkephalin in cultural peripheral blood mononuclear cells from patients infected with human immunodeficiency virus. Clin Immunol Immunopathol 51:386–395, 1989

Olschowka JA, O'Donohue TL, Mueller GP, et al: The distribution of corticotropin releasing factor-like immunoreactivity neurons in rat brain. Peptides 3:995–1015, 1982a

Olschowka JA, O'Donohue TL, Mueller GP, et al: Hypothalamic and extrahypothalamic distribution of CRF-like immunoreaction neurons in the rat brain. Neuroendocrinology 35:305–308, 1982b

Padgett GA, Reiquam CW, Henson JB, et al: Comparative studies of susceptibility to infection in the Chediak-Higashi syndrome. J Pathol Bacteriol 95:509–522, 1968

Parker CW, Huber MG, Baumann ML: Alterations of the cyclic AMP metabolism in human bronchial asthma, III: leukocyte and lymphocyte responses to steroids. J Clin Invest 52:1342–1348, 1973

Parrillo JE, Fauci AS: Comparison of the effector cells in human spontaneous cellular cytotoxicity and antibody-dependent cellular cytotoxicity: differential sensitivity of effector cells to in vivo and in vitro corticosteroids. Scand J Immunol 8:99–107, 1978

Paul WE: The immune system: an introduction, in Fundamental Immunology. Edited by Paul WE. New York, Raven, 1984, pp 3–22

Plotnikoff NP, Miller GC, Solomon S, et al: Methionine-enkephalin: immunomodulator in normal volunteers (in vivo). Psychopharmacol Bull 22:1097–1100, 1986a

Plotnikoff NP, Wybran J, Nimeh NF, et al: Methionine-enkephalin: enhancement of T-cells in patients with Kaposi's sarcoma (AIDS). Psychopharmacol Bull 22:695–697, 1986b

Puppo F, Corsini G, Mangini P, et al: Influences of β-endorphin on phytohemagglutinin-induced lymphocyte proliferation and on the expression on mononuclear cell surface antigens in vitro. Immunopharmacology 10:119–125, 1985

Riley V: Psychoneuroendocrine influences on immunocompetence and neoplasia. Science 212:1100–1109, 1981

Ritz J: The role of natural killer cells in immune surveillance. N Engl J Med 320:1748–1749, 1989

Rivier C, Vale W, Ling N: Stimulation in vivo of the secretion of prolactin and growth hormone by β-endorphin. Endocrinology 100:238–241, 1977

Schleifer SJ, Keller SE, Camerino M, et al: Suppression of lymphocyte stimulation following bereavement. J Am Med Assoc 250:374–377, 1983

Schleifer SJ, Keller SE, Meyerson AT, et al: Lymphocyte function in major depressive disorder. Arch Gen Psychiatry 41:484–486, 1985

Schleifer SJ, Keller SE, Bond RN, et al: Major depressive disorder and immunity: role of age, sex, severity, and hospitalization. Arch Gen Psychiatry 46:81–87, 1989

Selye H: Stress in Health and Disease. Boston, MA, Butterworth, 1976

Shavit Y, Lewis JW, Terman GW, et al: Opioid peptides mediate the suppressive effect of stress on natural killer cell cytotoxicity. Science 223:188–190, 1984

Shavit Y, Terman GW, Martin FC, et al: Stress, opioid peptides, the immune system, and cancer. J Immunol 135:8340–8370, 1985

Shavit Y, Depaulis A, Martin FC, et al: Involvement of brain opiate receptors in the immune-suppressive effect of morphine. Proc Natl Acad Sci USA 83:7114–7117, 1986a

Sherman JE, Kalin NH: ICV-CRH potently affects behavior without altering antinociceptive responding. Life Sci 39:433–441, 1985

Sibinga NES, Goldstein A: Opioid peptides and opioid receptors in cells of the immune system. Ann Rev Immunol 6:219–249, 1988

Strom TD, Lundin AP, Carpenter CB: Role of cyclic nucleotides in lymphocytes activation and function. Prog Clin Immunol 3:115–153, 1977

Sullivan JL, Byron KS, Brewster FE, et al: Deficient natural killer activity in X-linked lymphoproliferative syndrome. Science 210:543–545, 1980

Sutton RE, Koob GF, LeMoal M, et al: Corticotropin releasing factor produces behavioral activation in rats. Nature 297:331–333, 1982

Swanson LW, Sawchenko PE, Rivier J, et al: The organization of ovine corticotropin releasing factor (CRF). Neuroendocrinology 36:165–186, 1983

Taylor AI, Fishman LM: Corticotropin releasing hormone. N Engl J Med 319:213–222, 1988

Trinchieri G: Biology of natural killer cells. Adv Immunol 47:187–376, 1989

Urich A, Muller C, Aschaver H, et al: Lytic effector cell function in schizophrenia and depression. J Neuroimmunol 18:291–301, 1988

Vale W, Spiess J, Rivier C, et al: Characterization of a 41-residue ovine hypothalamic peptide that stimulates secretion of corticotropin and beta-endorphin. Science 213:1394–1397, 1981

Valentino RJ, Foote SL, Aston-Jones G: CRF activates noradrenergic neurons of the locus coeruleus. Brain Res 270:363–367, 1983

Van Loon GR, Appel NM: β-endorphin-induced hyperglycemia is mediated by increased central sympathetic outflow to adrenal medulla. Brain Res 204:236–241, 1981

Von Euler US: The presence of a substance with sympathin E properties in spleen extracts. Acta Physiol Scand 11:168–170, 1946

Watson JJ: The influence of intracellular levels of cyclic nucleotides on cell proliferation and the induction of antibody synthesis. J Exp Med 141:97–111, 1975

Weber RJ, Pert A: The periaqueductal gray matter mediates opiate-induced immunosuppression. Science 245:188–190, 1989

Webster EL, de Souza EB: Corticotropin releasing factor receptors in mouse spleen: identification, autoradiographic localization, and regulation by divalent cations and guanim nucleotides. Endocrinology 122:609–617, 1988

Webster EL, Tracey DE, Jutila MA, et al: Corticotropin releasing factor receptors in mouse spleen: identification of receptor-bearing cells as resident macrophages. Endocrinology 127:440–452, 1990

Weiss JM, Goodman PA, Losito BG, et al: Behavioral depression produced by an uncontrollable stressor: relationship to norepinephrine, dopamine, and serotonin levels in various regions of rat brain. Brain Research Reviews 3:167–205, 1981

Williams LT, Snyderman R, Lefkowitz RJ: Identification of beta-adrenergic receptors in human lymphocytes by (-)3H-alprenolol binding. J Clin Invest 57:149–155, 1976

Wybran J, Appelboom T, Famaey JP, et al: Suggestive evidence for receptors for morphine and methionine-enkephalin on normal human blood T lymphocytes. J Immunol 123:1068–1072, 1979

Wybran J, Schandene L, Van Vooren JP, et al: Immunologic properties of methionine enkephalin, and therapeutic implications in AIDS, ARC, and cancer. Ann NY Acad Sci 496:108–114, 1987

Wynn PC, Hauger RL, Holmes MC: Brain and pituitary receptors for corticotropin releasing factor's localization and differential regulation after adrenalectomy. Peptides 5:1077–1084, 1984

Zinkernagel RM, Doherty PC: MHC-restricted cytotoxic T cells: studies on the biological role of polymorphic major transplantation antigens determining T-cell restriction-specificity, function, and responsiveness, in Advances in Immunology. New York, Academic, 1979, pp 51–177

Zunich KM, Kirkpatrick CH: Methionine-enkephalin as immunomodulator therapy in human immunodeficiency virus infections: clinical and immunological effects. J Clin Immunol 8:95–102, 1988